Interviewing and Counseling in Communicative Disorders

PRINCIPLES AND PROCEDURES

SECOND EDITION

Kenneth G. Shipley
California State University, Fresno

Allyn and Bacon

Boston London Toronto Sydney Tokyo Singapore

Copyright © 1997, 1992 by Allyn & Bacon
A Viacom Company
Needham Heights, MA 02194

Library of Congress Cataloging-in-Publication Data

Shipley, Kenneth G.
    Interviewing and counseling in communicative disorders : principles and procedures / Kenneth G. Shipley ; with a chapter contributed by Celeste Roseberry-McKibbin. — 2nd ed.
        p.   cm.
    Includes bibliographical references and index.
    ISBN 0-205-19892-9
    1. Counseling. 2. Interviewing.   I. Roseberry-McKibbin, Celeste.
II. Title.
BF637.C6S52   1996
616.85´5--dc20   96-7010
                                                                  C I P

Printed in the United States of America
10 9 8 7 6 5 4 3 2 1   00 99 98 97 96

Contents

Preface to the Second Edition

The purpose of this book is to describe the fundamentals of effective interviewing and counseling in speech-language pathology and audiology. To accomplish this purpose, I have tried to integrate a variety of literature on interviewing and counseling, along with my experience providing clinical services, supervising clinical practicum, and teaching a variety of courses in communicative disorders, including interviewing and counseling classes. The basic principles and procedures of interviewing and counseling and the specific techniques and suggestions in this book are applicable to children and adults, to clients and caregivers, and to all settings in which clinicians provide service.

Professionals working with communicative disorders have long recognized the importance of effective interviewing and counseling skills in clinical activities. Yet, as many authorities and clinicians have lamented for years, interviewing and counseling is a neglected area within most professional education programs. A large number of graduates go into the clinical and educational services workplace with neither coursework nor effective practicum experiences in these areas. Too often, clinicians must learn how to interview and counsel on their own, in a "hit-and-miss" fashion, while on the job. Learning such essential skills this way is difficult for clinicians and is a disservice to many clients. Also, such a method of learning does not necessarily mean that the most effective methods of interviewing and counseling are discovered along the way.

This book is designed for use by students or professionals working with communicative disorders. The first edition was used as both a primary and secondary text in many communicative disorders courses. It was used in undergraduate and graduate-level courses dealing with interviewing and counseling, in assessment and diagnostics courses, and in clinical methods coursework. The book also was used with clinical practica, in internships, and in student teaching. Professionals, particularly those who never had specific coursework or practica in interviewing and counseling, found that it addressed a wide range of pertinent, practical topics. This second edition should be useful in these same ways; it treats a variety of situations clinicians face and describes methods and techniques applicable to students as well as professionals.

I have tried to organize the book for easy reading and reference. There are eleven chapters; two of them have appendices. Three additional appendices, the references, and an index are at the back of the book.

Chapter 1 provides an overview of interviewing and counseling and its uses. Also introduced are some of the basic methods clinicians use to obtain information. Chapters 2, 3, and 4 address the prerequisites of effective interviewing and counseling, the factors that influence communication in interviewing and counseling situations, and the skills and techniques clinicians need to recognize and develop to become effective interviewers and counselors. A number of conditions and behaviors that impact clinical interviews are considered in these chapters. Effective clinicians use many of the skills, techniques, and behaviors discussed here to promote success when interviewing and counseling.

Then, Chapters 5, 6, and 7 address the specific purposes, structure, and content of information-getting and information-giving interviews and of counseling activities. These chapters describe the interactions in which clinicians obtain information; provide information; provide support to clients; help clients release counterproductive feelings; or try to teach, influence, persuade, or counsel others. A number of techniques and suggestions to achieve effective interactions with patients, their families, or other caregivers are included in each of these chapters.

A number of cross-cultural considerations and factors that influence interviewing and counseling sessions are addressed throughout the book. In addition, Chapter 8 specifically addresses multicultural practice in relation to interviewing and counseling. Dr. Celeste Roseberry-McKibbin, a well-known authority on multicultural practice in communicative sciences and disorders, a colleague, and a valued friend, has kindly contributed this chapter. Her contribution is an important addition to the second edition.

Chapter 9 covers a wide range of potentially difficult-to-deal-with circumstances interviewers and counselors encounter in their practice. Topics in this chapter range from encountering anger and hostility, to working with certain types of defensive behavior and defense mechanisms, to helping patients who are experiencing grief or are in the midst of a crisis. Chapter 10 deals with a number of ethical, procedural, and professional matters that affect interviewing and counseling activities. Many of these topics are discussed in relation to the Code of Ethics of the American Speech-Language-Hearing Association.

Chapter 11 contains a few final thoughts, particularly about learning to interview and counsel and about increasing one's skills in these areas. The fundamentals of effective interviewing and counseling, and practical suggestions and techniques are offered throughout the book. Several checklists for learning and self-evaluating particular skills are found in several chapters. The appendices in Chapter 7 are two methods that can be used to evaluate counseling sessions.

The literature on interviewing and counseling in communicative disorders is rather sparse, but there is a large body of information available from disciplines such as counseling, psychology, social work, education, and even medicine. Thus many of the fundamental principles and techniques addressed here are drawn from those fields as they apply to our disciplines.

One thing that readers will not find in *Interviewing and Counseling in Communicative Disorders* is a focus on particular communicative disorders. Different disorders are mentioned in various places, but readers will not find specific sections on how to interview or counsel clients who are stuttering, who have had a laryngectomy, who are experiencing a hearing loss, and so forth. Rather, this work focuses on how to interview and counsel effectively across disorders because the interviewing fundamentals "cut across" particular disorders, age levels, and settings of practice. The precise content areas for interviewing and counseling with different disorders are easily adaptable into these basic skills. For example, students and professionals can draw on information from their coursework and experience with different types of articulation, fluency, hearing, language, and voice problems and directly apply this to their interviewing and counseling activities.

Acknowledgments

It is not possible to properly acknowledge all the individuals—colleagues, teachers, students, clients and their families and caregivers, and friends—who have knowingly or unknowingly contributed to the first and now the second edition of this book. I do, though, wish to express my gratitude to the following people.

Dr. Kenneth W. Burk, Professor of Communicative Disorders and Sciences at Wichita State University, spawned my interest in interviewing and counseling. Jeanne Hagen Stoddard, a very special student and now an exceptional speech-language pathologist, was immensely helpful in spawning my interest in writing the first edition and assisting with some of the research for that edition. Julie G. McAfee, my graduate research assistant for the first edition and now a successful speech-language pathologist and my coauthor on a different book, did a superb job of helping with research and manuscript preparation on the first edition. Her good work and insightful questions continued to be felt when writing this edition.

Christine Maul and Teresina Ramariz served as primary assistants with the current edition. Their help was outstanding and is truly appreciated. Erin Stevens and Glen Tellis also provided very useful help within several specific areas of the book.

Dr. Celeste Roseberry-McKibbin merits special appreciation. She very willingly contributed a valuable chapter on multicultural practice (see Chapter 8), and also assisted in reviewing and making suggestions throughout the book. Her contribution makes a valuable impact on the second edition.

I also appreciate the help and support of the highly skilled staff at Allyn and Bacon and its consultants, including Dr. Roberta De Pompei of the University of Akron, School of Communicative Disorders, Akron, Ohio; Dr. Peter Feudo, Jr., of Marywood College, Department of Communication Sciences and Disorders, Scranton, Pennsylvania; and Dr. Candis Warner of Western Michigan University, Department of Speech Pathology and Audiology, Kalamazoo, Michigan. Special thanks are also extended to my editor, Kris Farnsworth, who sought this second edition and was always helpful during its development and publication; and to Marilyn Rash of Ocean Publication Services who edited the final text and coordinated the production details.

Appreciation is also extended for the assistance and support of the Research Committee of the School of Health and Human Services at California State University, Fresno, and to my dean, Dr. Benjamin Cuellar. Their help was invaluable in helping expedite the preparation process. My students and colleagues in the Department of Communicative Sciences and Disorders also assisted in many ways, from their supportive comments to understanding why I was not at my desk quite as often as normal while working on this edition.

Finally, my loving appreciation goes to Peggy and Jennifer, whose patience did not falter and who put up with some very divided attention. I love and thank you both!

Chapter *1*

Interviewing and Counseling in the Clinical Process

Interviewing and counseling are extremely important activities for clinicians working with people experiencing speech, language, or hearing disorders (Clark, 1994a; Haynes, Pindzola, & Emerick, 1992; McFarlane, Fujiki, & Brinton, 1984; Neidecker & Blosser, 1993, Stone & Olswang, 1989; Taylor, 1992). To illustrate this, consider the following comments:

> *Of all the skills required for speech clinicians, there are none so important as the skills needed for interviewing, taking case histories, and counseling. Everything else we do depends upon how well these are done.* (Hutchinson, 1979, p. 1)

> *Although clinical evaluation obviously involves more than proficiency at conducting interviews, this skill is central to the role of the diagnostician. By means of verbal exchange, we gather information about the individual, transmit information, and establish a working relationship. The interview is also the means by which treatment is carried out and, as such, serves both as a tool and as a relationship. For the clinical speech-language pathologist, interviewing is an extremely important activity.* (Haynes et al., 1992, p. 29)

> *The ability to talk to people—to skillfully and systematically divine the important aspects of a voice disorder and then counsel appropriately—is a skill that must be mastered . . . The initial patient interview and subsequent counseling are the most important aspects of a voice evaluation.* (Stemple, 1993, p. 172)

> *Counseling is a recognized and vital component to the intervention services that we provide to our patients. To be most effective in serving patients and their families, audiologists must become adept not only in the diagnosis of auditory disorders and the rehabilitative management of these disorders, but also in the more elusive area of successful patient-professional relationships that may be built and maintained through the art of counseling.* (Clark, 1994a, pp. 2-3)

These are just four examples from many that could have been included here, because it is well recognized that interviewing and counseling activities are vitally important for effectively delivering services in speech-language pathology and audiology. The need for effective interviewing and counseling cuts across types of disorders, severity of disorders, settings, age groups, and cultural backgrounds.

Despite the general acceptance of interviewing and counseling as necessary and important for effective practice, preprofessional coursework and practice within these areas is woefully inadequate (Clark, 1994a; Colton & Casper, 1990; Culpepper, Mendel, & McCarthy, 1994; Johnson, 1994). Many professionals have little or no coursework in the areas of interviewing and counseling, and only minimal preprofessional clinical practicum dealing specifically in these areas. Thus, many practitioners begin their careers with some fear of interviewing and counseling as they learn these skills by "trial and error." This type of learning sometimes occurs at the expense of several patients along the way. This is, indeed, unfortunate and certainly not in the best interests of either clinicians or those they serve.

The following sections address some of the basic information-gathering techniques used in diagnostic and assessment activities. The three basic types of interviews—information-getting interviews; information-giving interviews; and persuasive, influencing, or counseling interviews—are then introduced. This is followed by some of the basic principles of learning or improving interviewing and counseling skills and abilities.

Methods of Obtaining Information

All clinical treatment services—from providing one-to-one intervention, to group treatment, to implementing home or classroom activities, to dispensing amplification devices—are based on a clinician's understanding of their client's specific communicative abilities and needs. This understanding begins developing as clinicians gain information from their client or from others who are familiar with a client (parents, significant others, caregivers, adult children, teachers, physicians). Clinicians typically gain a majority of their initial information from case history questionnaires, interviews, and, when available, written reports from other professionals who have worked with the client (Shipley &

McAfee, 1992). Clinicians gain further information from direct observation and direct evaluation of different communicative skills.

A clinician's evaluation of a patient typically culminates in identifying the presence or absence of a problem. If a problem exists, a diagnosis, an estimate of prognosis, and a plan of action or treatment are developed. These types of information are subsequently shared with clients or their caregivers in an information-giving interview. This entire process of collecting the case history; observing and evaluating the client's communicative abilities and needs; determining a diagnosis, prognosis, and plan of action; and sharing these determinations occurs within one appointment in some settings and with some cases. In other settings or with more complex cases, this process may occur over several occasions during several days or even a couple of weeks.

Case History Questionnaires

A questionnaire is a written form of a case history. Clients, or their parents or other caregivers, are asked to identify and describe various factors that may relate to a communicative disorder. Common areas of inquiry on case history forms include speech, language, motor skills; and family, social, medical, educational, or other appropriate histories. Three examples of case history forms are in Appendices A, B, and C.

Written case histories should be viewed as "starting points" for further investigation and inquiry. By their very nature, case histories have some inherent limitations. According to Shipley and McAfee (1992), several of these are:

1. Respondents may not understand some of the terminology used on the form so incomplete or inaccurate information results.
2. There may be insufficient time to complete the entire form, or think about answers for information requested.
3. Respondents may not know, or only have a vague recall of, some information requested.
4. Significant amounts of time may have gone by between the onset of problems and the current assessment.
5. Other events or circumstances, either at present or in the past, may hinder the recall of certain information.
6. Cultural differences, or difficulties with the language, may interfere with providing certain information.

In many settings, respondents complete the written case history form and return it beforehand, or bring it with them to the first visit. Other service providers supply the written case history form to clients at the first visit; it is then completed before an assessment session or during an initial interview. These variations are based on policies and perceived needs of professionals who work at the different settings.

One advantage of having a written history completed before the first visit is that the client and/or other informant may be able to supply more reliable information regarding the speech, language, hearing, medical, academic, social, or other appropriate histories. This gives people a chance to think about the questions asked and determine what information is being requested in private (Martin, 1994). The individual completing the form can also talk with family members, teachers, or other persons who can provide additional information regarding any specifics sought.

Another advantage of having a case history form completed beforehand is that time can be saved during an initial visit. Having already collected and reviewed the basic case history information, clinicians have a starting point and some sense of the most important areas that need to be discussed. Preliminary information about the problem and its progression can then be further explored, expanded on, and validated during the initial interview. When a diagnostic session is scheduled on the same day, having the case history completed and returned in advance allows clinicians to prepare for the assessment session. Knowing such details as the client's age and gender and having someone's perceptions of the problem can help clinicians select appropriate materials, including formal or informal test procedures, or prepare in other ways for the diagnostic session.

There are, however, several potential disadvantages to having the case history completed and returned before the first visit. Emerick and Haynes (1986) note some settings use "generic" or "universal" questionnaires—that is, the same form is used for many disorder types. Generic forms cannot address all the information needed for specific types of disabilities (for fluency, voice, articulation, and so forth). Most settings do have separate forms for children and adults, but these forms may not adequately distinguish the differences between age levels with children. There are, for example, important differences between infants and toddlers, and between preschool-, elementary school-, junior high and high school-age children.

One way to overcome part of the problem of generic forms is to use a generic case history for basic information and a second, more specific history form that focuses on particular communicative disorders (fluency, hearing impairment, early childhood language, aphasia, and so forth). Appendix B contains an example of a disorder-specific questionnaire developed for use with the area of voice.

Another potential disadvantage of having the case history completed beforehand is that there may be some questionnaire items—particularly those dealing with prenatal and birth experiences, medical history, and communicative development—that may cause some informants to feel threatened or guilty. Sometimes, such reactions are discovered during an initial interview; other times, such reactions are not shared with clinicians.

Supplying a case history before a first visit can cause other problems. Informants may not understand certain questions or may misinterpret them. As a result, inaccurate or incomplete information is provided. Also, people with poor reading and writing skills may be unable to complete the form, may accidentally supply inaccurate or incomplete information, or may become embarrassed or intimidated by their inabilities. Completing case history forms can be very difficult and frustrating for some multicultural clients who do not have adequate skills in the language used on the form or are unsure why certain questions need to be asked. In such cases, it is wise to complete the form together with the client. Having the case history form available in different languages is useful in some settings.

Completing a case history form with clients is time-consuming, and it can prevent the participants from interacting freely and naturally with each other. The scope of discussions may be restricted to those topics covered by the case history form. Further, an informant may not be sufficiently prepared to give complete and accurate answers to the various questions asked on the form.

In summary, there is no perfect answer to having case history forms completed beforehand or with the clinician; rather, circumstances surrounding the case and the setting may dictate which approach works best. In general, my suggestion is to provide respondents with the case history form before the first visit. The form can be accompanied by a request to provide the information that is known, and an indication that any questions will also be discussed during the first meeting. This gives the client/informant an opportunity to ponder the questions asked and to find any information that is not readily accessible from memory. Any answers that are incomplete or need further clarification and discussion can then be reviewed with the client during the first visit.

Observation

Observing behavior is an important technique for obtaining information and insight. Observation plays an important role in assessment as well as treatment activities. Darley (1978) outlines two basic types of observational approaches: spectator observation and participant observation. *Spectator observation* occurs when an observer is physically removed or apart from the client and the situation being observed. The clinician may or may not be out of sight of the client or out of the room; if the clinician is out of sight, the observation may take place through a one-way mirror, by video monitor, in a classroom, or even on a playground. Presumably, such observations produce objective, firsthand information because communicative behavior can be observed unobtrusively. However, the range of behaviors, and even the types of communicative interactions available for observation, can be limited in many settings. For example, clients are most frequently observed in a clinical or educational setting where their behavior can differ, sometimes considerably, from what might be seen in more typical environments. Thus, the communicative behaviors or interactions observed may not be representative of an individual's normal functioning.

The second type of observation is participant observation, which is used frequently in speech-language pathology and audiology. *Participant observations* allow clinicians to structure situations to elicit specific responses or behaviors. Standardized testing is one form of participant observation. Another form is a speech-language sample in which clinicians observe and record samples of an individual's actual communicative skills.

A disadvantage of participant observation is the potential influence that clinicians themselves and their presentation of tasks can have on a client's behavior. In effect, what is presented by the clinician may dictate what is actually observed. Or, the very structure of the situation, like the setting for the spectator observation, may not be conducive to eliciting representative samples of the client's communicative behavior. Despite these potential variables, participant observations typically provide valuable information about clients, their families or other caregivers, basic patterns of interacting, and actual communicative skills and needs.

A clinician's observations are typically focused on how well the client speaks, hears, comprehends, and uses language. The clinician may also try to judge a client's level of comfort within the setting, as well as the client's general attitudes toward the communicative problems. When a client's family members or caregivers are present, the interactive relationship between the client and those persons is frequently observed. Both what is said and how it is said may be important. For example, is a parent's speech and language use appropriate for the child? Does the spouse seem to dominate the interaction? Do the individuals appear to get along? These are only three examples of the kinds of dynamics the clinician can observe to gain information and insight.

As Mowrer (1988) comments:

> *Observation of behavior plays a major role towards our understanding of why humans behave the way they do. Yet, how we observe, what we observe, where we observe, when we observe, and what we do with the observation is . . . a very complex process.* (p. 60)

Good observational skills increase with concentration and practice. Skilled observers are able to see, hear, and sense specific details in a client's behavior or interactive style that a less sophisticated observer is likely to miss. Skilled observers are also able to distinguish relevant from irrelevant details in order to develop an understanding of the individual and the communicative problem.

Interviews

The case history questionnaire and a clinician's preliminary observations can provide information that sets a stage for any interactions that follow. The questionnaire may or may not be completed before the first interview, but either way, the clinician will have an opportunity to address and clarify areas of concern revealed on the case history form, or by observation, during an initial interview. During the interview, new information can emerge about the origin, course, and present state of the problem as well as about the client's or informant's feelings and attitudes about problems experienced. The information gathered during the initial interview, together with the information from an assessment session, will become the foundation for determining a diagnosis, prognosis, and treatment recommendations.

Definition of Interviews

An interview is a serious conversation conducted for one or more important purposes. It is a communicative event between someone with specific knowledge or expertise in an area and someone who would presumably benefit from that expertise. Dillard and Reilly (1988a) note that there are three significant dimensions to an interview: a purpose, a plan of action, and good communication. Inadequacy in any of these dimensions precludes optimal effectiveness in an interview.

Interviewing is a process of "dyadic communication" with a predetermined and serious purpose (Shipley & Wood, 1996; Stewart & Cash, 1994). A *dyad* is a form of interpersonal communication involving person-to-person interactions in which pervasive feedback occurs between two parties. There may be more than two people involved in a dyad, but there are never more than two parties involved—an interviewer party and an interviewee party. For example, when an entire family interacts with one interviewer, the two parties to the dyad are the family and the interviewer.

Fenlason (1962) suggests that a predetermined purpose distinguishes the interview from other types of conversations. Communication in a communicative disorders interview is designed to focus on specific matters, which are typically the client's communicative development, abilities and disabilities, and needs.

Unique Aspects of Interviewing and Counseling Activities

Stewart and Cash's (1994) excellent book, *Interviewing: Principles and Practices,* contains considerable information on the uniqueness and usefulness of interviews. Some of the information in this section is based on their work.

Besides being useful for obtaining basic facts, interviews provide information about people's feelings, thoughts, attitudes, and beliefs. Interviews tend to focus on personal needs or problems, whereas other communicative events (a cordial conversation, a speech, a lecture) operate within less sensitive, less personal areas of discussion. Another characteristic of interviews is that they encourage the use of various kinds and types of questions. Interviews are also unique in that, for a variety of reasons, digressions occur and should be expected. In fact, digressions into areas of previous discussion are often both necessary and planned. But in contrast to such communicative events as a speech or a lecture, in which a speaker can plan exactly what to say, the give-and-take nature of an interview does not afford the luxury of even knowing all areas of discussion that may arise.

There is an element of personal risk for both parties during interviewing and counseling activities. Clients, for example, risk being judged as doing the wrong thing; appearing to be a poor parent, spouse, or caregiver; revealing something that might later be regretted; or appearing to be weak or uninformed. Clinicians, meanwhile, risk not knowing the answers to certain questions, responding inappropriately, or appearing novice-like or inadequate. These risks are one reason some beginning clinicians are fearful of interviewing and, to an even greater degree, of counseling. These areas of risk also help explain why even more experienced clinicians may enter into certain interviewing and counseling activities with some degree of anxiety or uncertainty.

Types of Interviews

An interview regarding a communicative disorder is typically held for one of three reasons: (1) to secure information; (2) to provide information; or (3) to influence or alter someone else's feelings, attitudes, or behaviors. Thus, depending on its purpose, an interview may be one of three different types: (1) an information-getting interview; (2) an information-giving interview; or (3) an influencing, persuading, or counseling interview (Shipley & Wood, 1996). For example, if a clinician is trying to determine what factors are contributing to a speech or hearing problem, an *information-getting* interview is in order. If the clinician is describing assessment results, sharing suggested treatment options, or providing ongoing feedback regarding progress in treatment, an *information-giving* interview is conducted. If the clinician is involved in trying to assuage, modify, or alter someone's activities or feelings, a *counseling* type of interview is used. Of course, any given interview often involves a combination of these functions. For example, a clinician may have completed a diagnostic session and be involved primarily with providing information about the findings (information-giving) but, during the same session, continues to seek additional information deemed necessary (information-getting). Similarly, some information-getting interviews conducted primarily to obtain information also may involve helping people vent frustrations, or to persuade or counsel.

The following sections contain an overview of the three major types of interviewing and counseling activities. Chapters 5, 6, and 7 contain more complete discussions of these three basic types of interactions.

Information-Getting

Information-getting interviews are important in communicative disorders because the basic information obtained from clients, their caregivers, or other professionals can be a key to diagnosis and to remedial planning (Haynes et al., 1992; Peterson & Marquardt, 1994; Shipley & McAfee, 1992). Thus, information-getting interviews are, or should be, a routine part of the assessment or diagnostic process in all settings. During this type of interview the clinician may seek objective information such as dates or specific conditions and events that preceded a communicative difficulty; and the clinician may seek subjective information such as the interviewee's interpretations, attitudes, and feelings about the problems being experienced.

An information-getting interview is often the first interaction between a clinician and client or the client's family or caregivers. As the initial contact, an information-getting interview is the foundation on which the client–clinician relationship begins to develop. Thus, appropriate approaches and techniques for gathering information are vitally important. This type of interview is also conducted with people who are enrolled for ongoing services; for example, to determine whether newly learned behavior is generalizing into other situations or to other people, to learn results of some medical, educational, or psychological testing done elsewhere, and so forth.

Information-Giving

Clinicians are frequently involved in providing information to others. Test results, diagnostic impressions, suggestions, and recommendations may need to be conveyed to clients, their families or caregivers, or even to other professionals. Following diagnostic sessions, clinicians typically provide information concerning the nature of a communicative difficulty, any prognostic implications, and a proposed plan for case management. Information-giving interviews also occur in the course of treatment. For example, conscientious clinicians use this type of interview, even if they are somewhat informal, to provide feedback to clients and their families regarding treatment progress.

Providing information to others is important and, ultimately, the clinician must choose what type of information to provide and how to accurately convey it. When information is not provided well, clients or caregivers are likely to be confused, misinformed, or inadequately informed.

Counseling Activities

Counseling is a general term that embraces a number of clinical activities. When interviews are used to influence someone's behaviors or attitudes, they can be called helping, influencing, persuading, or counseling interviews (see Benjamin, 1981; Ivey, 1994; Shipley & Wood, 1996; Stewart & Cash, 1994). For purposes in this book, these types of interactions will usually be referred to as counseling interviews. In addition to altering behaviors or attitudes, counseling interviews are used to provide release, support, and encouragement for interviewees.

Audiologists and speech-language pathologists often see people with devastating communicative disorders that alter the lives of everyone surrounding their clients. In the case of acquired brain damage, for example, the disruption of communicative abilities can cause many major changes for the client and the client's family and friends. In such a case, a once-competent communicator experiences tremendous difficulties expressively, receptively, or both. The clinician serving such an individual will need to address a number of areas of everyday living with the client and with loved ones who are affected by the client's communicative disorder.

Through counseling, the clinician provides individuals with support and direction, and encourages the client and family members or caregivers to express important feelings and attitudes about the difficulties. The client's family members or caregivers may also be helped to modify their methods of interaction, to assist in treatment activities, or to understand and correct ways they may be hindering the client's progress. Similar types of examples, of course, are possible across a wide range of ages and disorder types.

Concluding Comments

The interview plays a significant role in the clinical process—obtaining information, providing information or teaching, helping people ventilate feelings and frustrations, and modifying behavior and attitudes. The foundation for a clinician's work is an understanding of a client that is developed from various sources of information—case history questionnaires, the initial information-getting interview, and direct observation during assessment sessions and at other times. A clinician's understanding is represented by a diagnosis, prognosis, and plans for remediation, which are usually shared in information-giving interviews. Although we have distinguished three different kinds of interviews—information-getting, information-giving, and counseling interviews—an actual interview at any time during the clinical process can involve any combination of the three functions.

Prerequisites for Effective Interviewing and Counseling

Effective interviewers and counselors possess an interest in others, know the field of communicative disorders, are able to provide appropriate counsel, and use a variety of techniques to facilitate communication. Successful clinicians also possess certain basic personal characteristics that facilitate effective communication with others.

Interviewer Characteristics

There are a number of personal attributes, attitudes, and beliefs that are characteristic of clinicians who perform interviewing and counseling functions well. The following pages describe some basic, prerequisite factors that contribute to working successfully with others. These fundamental attributes come from interviewing and counseling sources such as Biggs and Blocher (1987), DeBlassie (1976), Dillard and Reilly (1988b), Hackney and Cormier (1994), Moursund (1993), Okun (1992), Shertzer and Stone (1980), and Shipley and Wood (1996), and from the author's experiences conducting interviews and counseling in communicative disorders and teaching interviewing and counseling coursework.

Spontaneity. Clinicians need to be able to respond immediately and appropriately to situations and discussions that arise.

Flexibility.   Personal security, knowledge of the field and of people, and the abilities to be spontaneous are needed to be flexible. There is no single right or fixed way for all clinicians to interview or counsel; clinicians must vary their approaches when dealing with different clients, their families or caregivers, or others who often are involved.

Concentration.   Clinicians must be able to concentrate as completely as possible on what is occurring at all times during interactions with one or more individuals.

Openness.   Clinicians must be able to hear, understand, and accept the values and feelings of other people without distorting how they are feeling or what they are conveying. They also must be careful not to inappropriately impose their values on others.

Honesty.   Honesty is a key factor in developing trust and effective relationships. As Okun (1992) has commented, "honesty is more than just being truthful, it is also being open to exploration and being fair in evaluation" (p. 36).

Emotional stability.   Part of emotional stability involves security with self and the abilities to adapt to and flow with the experiences of life. Being in a helping profession is not always easy, so clinicians need to be emotionally stable and secure with themselves.

Trustworthiness.   Clinicians have little opportunity for success unless they are able to engender the trust of their clients, peers, and other professionals.

Self-awareness.   True self-awareness allows clinicians to understand their personal and professional strengths and weaknesses, the range and limitations of their abilities, and how others are responding to them. Clinicians must also be aware of their own biases and stereotypes regarding members of different linguistic, cultural, or religious backgrounds. It is important to be aware of any such biases or feelings they possess and not let these inappropriately influence clinical judgments.

Belief in people's ability to change.   Effective clinicians believe in change and in people's abilities to learn, to grow, and to change during the clinical process.

Commitment to people.   Deep commitments to people, to human values, and to the fulfillment of human potentials are important characteristics of effective clinicians.

Knowledge and wisdom. Clinicians need to be wise, knowledgeable, intellectually active, and inquisitive. They need to develop wisdom in their understanding of themselves, of others, of the world—and of the various conditions, experiences, skills, and techniques that promote optimal growth and self-actualization.

Good communicative skills. For interviewing and counseling, clinicians need good comprehension and listening skills, as well as good skills of expression. Good verbal and nonverbal communication skills are imperative; poor or tentative verbal skills significantly hamper clinical interactions. Similarly, using too few, too many, or incongruent nonverbal behaviors detract from clinical effectiveness.

Academic and clinical competence in speech-language pathology or audiology. Competence in the clinician's field of expertise is essential for interviewing and counseling to be effective. Without a solid understanding of the field, there is simply no basis for effectively working with people experiencing communicative difficulties.

These are some of the characteristics that make for effective interviewers and counselors. Such basic personality traits, personal feelings toward life, and individual attitudes are difficult for some people to acquire or control. But, clinicians do need to at least be aware of their personal qualities and the characteristics and attitudes they project. In some cases, the clinicians will have to modify counterproductive behavioral or attitudinal characteristics before they can provide services as effectively as possible.

Conditions That Facilitate Good Communication

Effective communication in interviewing and counseling situations depends on certain conditions being present in clinicians' and clients' relationships. These include sensitivity, respect, empathy, objectivity, listening skills, and motivation. When these elements are shared by the parties, rapport between the participants can be established and maintained.

Sensitivity

Sensitivity is important to professionals in all helping professions. Clinicians must realize that clients' feelings about a subject influence their thinking about and receptivity toward the topic of discussion. Their thinking may or may not be in accordance with a clinician's thoughts. For example, two parties may think differently about the "severity" of a problem; thus, an individual who is deeply embarrassed about having a mild lisp may be irritated by being told that the problem is "relatively minor." Conversely, parents who do not think that their child's problem is very severe often have difficulty understanding or agreeing with suggestions to the contrary. In both cases, a sensitive clinician will realize that personal perceptions and feelings about a subject will affect the individual's reactions toward any observations the specialist might share.

Clinicians need to be sensitive to their clients' interests in and levels of concern about their problems. Some clients or caregivers may be extremely concerned about a given problem; others may not be. At times, it can be difficult not to become annoyed with some clients' seemingly apathetic attitudes or statements. However, the clinicians' responsibility is to provide information and interpretations in straightforward, communicative fashions. When clinicians encounter a lack of interest or concern, they may need to objectively yet sensitively demonstrate why greater concern is warranted and to share the various ramifications of their findings.

There are certainly many factors related to sensitivity when interviewing or counseling across cultures. For example, some clinicians who were raised in a traditional, middle-class upbringing may find themselves becoming irritated when working with certain culturally or linguistically different individuals or families who appear apathetic toward a communicative disorder. Among some cultural groups, such as with some native Americans, a handicapped child may be accepted as a gift from the Great Spirit. Some other native American individuals believe that a child is born with a disability because the child chose prenatally to be disabled (Harris, 1993). Some Asians believe that disabilities and birth defects result from "sins" committed by parents or even remote ancestors; others believe that disabling conditions are that person's "fate" and that nothing should be done to interfere with this fate (Ethridge, 1990; Lewis & Vang, 1987). Certainly the clinician who does not recognize such cultural influences will be have difficulty with these sensitive issues when dealing with clients holding such views. Chapter 8 addresses a number of other factors related to cross-cultural sensitivity.

Sensitivity toward an interviewee's level of knowledge is also important. It is wise to remember that other people will not have had the years of training and clinical experience that a professional in communicative disorders has attained. Unless clinicians are sensitive in their use of language, and to the amount of knowledge other people have about communicative disorders, patients and caregivers can become misinformed or confused rather easily. Inappropriate assumptions about other people's knowledge of communicative difficulties and of technical terminology (e.g., terms like sibilant, impedance, prognosis, diadochokinesis, sensorineural) typically result in a failure to communicate effectively. Essentially, the client has no idea what the clinician is talking about or develops a mental picture that differs considerably from what the clinician intended to convey.

The use of technical jargon can also make the clinician appear insensitive, uncaring, or even arrogant (Enelow & Swisher, 1986); its use should be avoided whenever possible. Clinicians need to use simple, nontechnical language in their explanations and discussions. This is not to imply that they should avoid saying what needs to be said, or that clinicians should fall into the trap of providing false assurances. Rather, clinicians should balance their communication so that it is supportive as well as truthful. Sensitivity to clients' knowledge, background, and emotional-psychological state helps clinicians communicate effectively and promotes any changes deemed necessary.

Respect

Respect involves having regard for and showing appropriate courtesy to the other party. The words that clinicians use, as well as their actions and behaviors, act to convey respect or disrespect. Clinicians should share information cheerfully and respectfully (Mowrer, 1988). However, it is not always possible for the clinician to deliver "cheerful news"; in some situations, the clinician must be the bearer of bad news. For example, a clinician may need to convey to caregivers that their loved one has a serious communicative difficulty, that a neurological examination should be obtained, that a child cannot hear, that limited recovery will be possible, or that special education or special care should be considered.

Clearly, it is not appropriate to deliver all news cheerfully. It is possible, however, to help individuals see the positive aspects of any difficult-to-face information and to help them move ahead constructively. The clinician should respect the individual, the individual's feelings, and the individual's reactions to the information that must be faced.

As a matter of respect and sensitivity, clinicians should keep in mind the possibility that some interviewees and counselees will pose questions or concerns that, in a strict clinical sense, do not seem particularly important or even appropriate. However, it is a good guideline to assume that any question or concern posed by an interviewee is important to that person. Even seemingly irrelevant, "dumb," or repetitious questions should be handled forthrightly, courteously, and respectfully (Shipley & Wood, 1996).

Empathy

Empathy is defined here as the quality of being able to enter and share the feelings of others. In other words, the clinician truly feels and understands what the other person is feeling. Years ago, Fenlason (1962) commented that being able to identify with another person's feelings and actions "is the essence of understanding the *why* of another's attitudes and behavior" (p. 204). Empathy is built on caring attitudes, sensitivity, and knowledge and understanding of an individual's circumstances and feelings. During an interview, the clinician simultaneously learns about and attempts to understand the individual.

The verbal and nonverbal exchanges that occur in interviews are reflections of the participants' conscious intentions to communicate certain information, as well as the unconscious processes that may be going on in their minds. These unconscious aspects influence people's feelings and attitudes about an interaction. Again, interviewers need to be aware that their own attitudes create impressions and engender feelings and reactions. Skill in using various techniques is certainly no substitute for having appropriate attitudes toward interviewing, and empathy toward people in general. Techniques can be adopted to address a problem at hand, but in order to use these techniques properly, clinicians must be able to empathetically evaluate an interviewee's attitudes and personality. This requires considerable skill in human relations and caring attitudes.

Objectivity

Speech-language pathologists and audiologists involved with interviewing and counseling must remain objective in their clinical roles. However, objectivity does not mean being impersonal, unfriendly, or insensitive. It simply means that a clinician does not allow personal emotions to inappropriately influence the situation. A realistic and practical point of view can be maintained when interviewers remain objective. A lack of objectivity is one indication that clinicians are concentrating on their own feelings rather than on the feelings of their clients.

Successful interviewing requires the use of the somewhat conflicting attitudes of empathy and objectivity (Rich, 1968). It is important for clinicians to understand the difference between subjective and objective information and reactions. And, it is important to understand how clients can affect clinicians' behavior.

A clinician's role is not to judge others in a negative sense but to understand potential causes and sources of behavior and feelings. The clinician must understand the distinction between being a friend and being friendly. There can be a delicate balance between being friendly and being a friend that requires careful judgment, particularly when working across cultures. For example, in the traditional Filipino value system, professionals are expected to be personable, subject to reciprocal influence and affiliation, and sensitive to a family's desire for emotional closeness (Chan, 1992a). Other cultures, such as the white, general U.S. culture, will expect friendliness but less of an emotionally close, friendlike role.

Interviewers and interviewees should strive to become cooperative co-workers or partners (Campbell, 1993; Schuyler & Rushmer, 1987), with clinicians maintaining the role of a director and guide within the relationship. In this role, clinicians need to appreciate their own degree of ego involvement in the interviewing and counseling activities. Every-one has the need to look and feel good, but, this should not occur at the expense of clients. Clinicians must hold interviewees' welfare in the highest regard; their own personal needs and issues are secondary.

Listening Skills

Listening is an essential ingredient in interviewing and counseling. It is a very purposeful activity that requires considerable concentration and skill. Careful listening allows clinicians to obtain or provide the infor-mation needed for effective service delivery. Listening also allows clini-cians to gain valuable insights into how patients think and feel about themselves and others, and how they perceive the information being discussed (Benjamin, 1981). Careful listening helps clinicians begin to understand an interviewee's goals, ambitions, aspirations, values, and basic philosophies, as well as the types of coping strategies or defense mechanisms that may be present. Careful and effective listening can also provide a therapeutic function, in that a clinician may be one of the first persons to understand the client's particular problem (Garrett, 1982). The clinician is often the first person to truly understand the magnitude, effects, and various implications surrounding a particular communicative disorder.

Effective listening is a skill. However, Mowrer (1988) suggests that speech-language pathologists in particular tend to be verbal people whose training has emphasized direct diagnosis and treatment. He notes that skillful listening in interviewing and counseling is not an "automatic response" for all clinicians. As Ivey (1994) comments, "You can't learn about the client if you are doing the talking!" (p. 24). Part of this prob-lem is related to the lack of formal preparation in interviewing and counseling within preprofessional programs. Audiologists and speech-language pathologists often have a considerable amount of training and experience in hearing how speech is produced, but they typically have far less training in other aspects of listening and understanding.

There are at least four critical factors in effective listening: concen-tration, active participation, comprehension, and objectivity (Barbara, 1958). *Concentration* requires hearing what is said, having patience, and removing any distractions from the interaction. Concentrate on the matters at hand—not other unrelated thoughts and concerns. *Active participation* requires that the clinician's mind remain ready, alert, open, flexible, and free from distraction. *Comprehension* involves hearing the surface messages as well as the underlying meanings that are conveyed. As noted earlier, *objectivity* requires that the clinician avoid inadvert-ently or inappropriately imposing personal feelings and attitudes on interviewees and what they may be expressing. All of these aspects of artful listening are relatively easy to acknowledge, but, they require a good deal of skill and discipline to implement!

Approaches to listening.   Stewart and Cash (1994) describe three basic types of listening approaches that interviewers and counselors can use: (1) listening for comprehension, (2) listening with empathy, and (3) listening for evaluation. *Listening for comprehension* is a method of receiving content that requires little feedback from the listener. The listener remains objective and perhaps even somewhat detached rather than critically analyzing or responding to the other person's comments. *Listening with empathy* goes beyond simply receiving messages and actually conveys understanding of what the client may be experiencing emotionally. Listening empathetically often involves providing comfort, warmth, and reassurance. Clinicians who listen with empathy try to put themselves "in the other person's shoes," to understand the other party, or to express their understanding of the other's situation. *Listening for evaluation* means trying to use the information received for some type of an evaluative conclusion.

To illustrate these fundamental types of listening approaches, suppose that someone promised to do something but then "ran out of time" and did not complete the task that was promised by a given time. During the explanation that followed, the individual who is *listening for comprehension* might be listening to obtain additional information about what had happened in order to understand more fully. The *listening for empathy* listener might be listening or even responding with empathy or sympathy (e.g., "You must have been overwhelmed"). The *listening for evaluation* listener might be awaiting additional information that would confirm or rule out the possibility of time-management problems, inadequate abilities to complete the task, and so forth. Clinicians need to recognize that these different types of listening exist and that, depending on the particular circumstances at hand, each of the three types of listening can be used. Clinicians should be able to use each type of listening effectively when it is needed.

Concentration.   Listening well requires good attending skills (Ivey, 1994). A clinician can convey an impression of good listening and attending with appropriate eye contact, a slightly forward body posture to indicate interest, hand gestures and body postures, and by providing appropriate verbal feedback to indicate that information is being heard and understood. However, there is more to good listening than simply appearing to hear what is being said.

Concentration on what other people are saying can be a difficult skill to learn. It does not come naturally to everyone. As Ivey (1983) comments:

Learning how to concentrate is an exercise in discipline. You can quickly tell how attentive you are as a listener if you use this simple device. The next time you listen to someone make a talk, throw away your pencil. When the talk is over, jot down an outline of the speaker's important points. At first, you may find that you have difficulty remembering anything without the aid of notes. But if you practice, you will soon be able to widen your span of attention and remember the gist of what you heard. If you listen in this manner, you are using your mind as a notebook and no longer need to depend on mechanical aids. (p. 43)

Ivey's comments are not included here to suggest that clinicians discard their pens, pencils, notepads, or tape recorders. Rather, the point is that concentration is a skill that can be acquired and improved in most cases.

All topics introduced, all information presented, and all questions posed by clients are potentially important. It is helpful if a clinician is ready to provide the rationale behind any area of inquiry in case the respondent questions its importance. Culatta and Goldberg (1995) point out that parents will be less likely to be offended by certain questions if they know why these questions are being asked. This can be very important with certain multicultural clients for whom an interviewer's question appears too personal or embarrassing (Anderson & Fenichel, 1989).

Clinicians should avoid becoming overstimulated by or emotionally involved with what an interviewee says. Emotionally loaded words, attitudes expressed, or particular positions taken should not be allowed to interfere with listening and understanding. Clinicians need to identify and recognize the types of words and attitudes that affect them emotionally so that their impact will be reduced when they are encountered in sessions. With emotions under control, clinicians should be able to attend carefully to what is being said, particularly with difficult or hard-to-deal-with information (Barker, 1971).

The clinician should listen to more than just the "basic facts" being expressed and realize that the feelings or reasons behind the facts are sometimes as important as, if not more important than, any particular pieces of information conveyed. Effective interviewers and counselors concentrate on an interaction and avoid being distracted. The clinician should ask for a clarification if something is missed or not understood; this is a considerably better option than becoming confused or not fully understanding something. A clinician also needs to make sure she or he understands any point the other party is making before commenting on it. These tenets are important in all interviewing and counseling situations. They are, of course, particularly salient in the presence of language barriers or when an interpreter is involved.

Listening and activity levels.   A different way to view the act of listening is to look at the degree of listening-versus-nonlistening in relation to the degree of activity-or-passivity of the listener. In his book, *Communicating with Parents of Exceptional Children: Improving*

Parent-Teacher Relationships, Kroth (1985) presents a model for looking at these factors and how they influence an interview (see Figure
2.1). The information in the figure applies to both clinicians and clients,
and it complements the other information on listening presented in this
chapter. Kroth's model is just one way of interpreting the degree of
listening and activity that occurs during interviewing and counseling
sessions. It should also be noted that the degree of a listener's listening
and activity can change at various times during an interview. In general,
some people may be active listeners, but their roles and actions at different times during an interview may vary between being passive and
active, between listening and not listening. Participants' activity levels
and their appearance while listening are also culturally relative so care
is needed when applying this model across cultures.

Someone who is operating in Quadrant A of Figure 2.1 is a generally passive person who is listening and, therefore, very much part of
the interaction. This person may exhibit a variety of nonverbal signals
(e.g., forward leaning of the body, smiling approval or understanding,
positive head nodding) which suggest that the material under discussion is being received and understood. For clinicians, assuming the

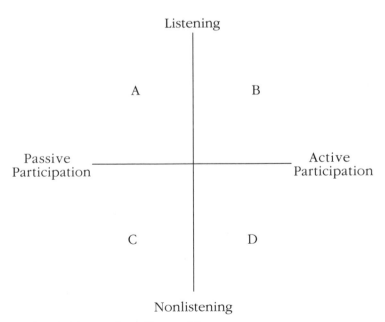

FIGURE 2.1   A Listening Paradigm

Source: From Roger L. Kroth, *Communicating with parents of exceptional children,*
2d ed. (p. 38). Copyright 1985 by and reprinted with permission of Love Publishing
Company, Denver, CO.

passive-listening role depicted in Quadrant A can sometimes be difficult if they usually take a more active role when interacting with clients.

Someone who is operating in Quadrant B is also listening attentively and is showing this in more active ways both verbally and nonverbally. Whoever is operating in Quadrant B—whether it is a clinician or a client—is very involved with active discussion. Clinicians may want to purposefully assume this active-listening role when they provide information to clients, or when they attempt to modify behavior or attitudes.

The participant in Quadrant C is a passive nonlistener. This person is neither listening nor active and is, therefore, rather difficult to work with. Little true communication occurs in interactions with this person. One person may be talking but little else is happening. The person in Quadrant C may very well hear what is said, while really being submerged in inner thought or resisting the information that is being provided.

Kroth (1985) describes and gives an example of passive nonlistening:

The passive nonlistener often seems to "hear" what is being said but is not involved in listening to the feeling content of the messages. This posture can be frustrating to the one who is trying to communicate with another person.

WIFE: *I'm so tired. I've been to four stores today trying to find material for a new dress. You're not listening!*

HUSBAND: *(folding the newspaper) You said you've been to four stores looking for material for a new dress.*

Although the content was accurate, the husband missed his wife's feelings of fatigue and frustration. She really could not argue that he was not listening, because he was able to parrot back most of her words accurately; however, no real communication took place. These are two people physically in the same room, one who is trying to send messages to alleviate some of her feelings and the other who is submerged in his own thoughts. (p. 39)

When I use this example with my classes, some married students share their feelings that their spouses are very capable of operating within Quadrant C. Dealing with Quadrant C clients can be very frustrating for clinicians because these people seem to hear the information while actually remaining distant from what is really being conveyed.

Finally, the participant in Quadrant D—the active nonlistener—is quite active within the encounter, but this person is not really listening to what is being conveyed. Effective communication is not occurring. Kroth (1985) presents the following example:

Almost everyone has had the experience of being at a social gathering where a great deal of talk was going on, with virtually no listening. In this type of conversation, people talk to each other but seldom with each other.

MRS. SMITH: *We're so glad you could come. I heard you were out of town.*

> MRS. JONES: *We just got back. We were attending my aunt's funeral in California.*
>
> MRS. SMITH: *California is so pretty this time of year. We were at Disneyland last spring. I enjoyed it so much.*
>
> MRS. JONES: *We were in Albuquerque last spring. Oh, there's Ruby. I must tell her about the squash-blossom necklace I found.* (p. 40)

This example is a little overstated from the point of view of most social interactions, but it does illustrate two people who are not listening to each other. When neither party in an interaction is listening, it is unlikely that either party will notice what is happening. In the case where one of the parties is listening but the other is not, communication will be one-sided at best. Kroth (1985) gives this example of one-sided active nonlistening at a parent-teacher conference:

> PARENT: *Billy had the neatest thing happen to him on his way home from school.*
>
> TEACHER: *How does he go home from school?*
>
> PARENT: *Down Center Street and —*
>
> TEACHER: *Isn't that past the fire station?*
>
> PARENT: *Yes, and—*
>
> TEACHER: *Last year five of our boys said they wanted to be firemen when they grow up. What does Billy want to be?*
>
> PARENT: *A nuclear physicist.*
>
> TEACHER: *Isn't that cute? And to think he can't even spell it. What happened to him on the way home?*
>
> PARENT: *Well, he ran into this man who—*
>
> TEACHER: *I hope he said "excuse me." We stress good manners in our room. We have a unit on the magic words—please and thank you. I hope you notice the improvement at home.* (p. 42)

Again, there is some overstatement in the example, but it does illustrate the idea of being verbally active but not listening.

It is important to remember how a participant's appearance of activity during an interview can belie the actual level of listening and receptivity. An important job of clinicians is to judge the other party's actual levels of listening and understanding that are occurring during an interview. It is also important for interviewers and counselors to understand their own characteristics of attending and listening. Figure 2.1 provides one model for self-assessment, or for estimating the listening and activity levels of others during interviewing or counseling sessions.

Of course, no one fits definitively into just one of the four quadrants. Individuals tend to operate within one of the quadrants more than in the others, but people may move into the other three quadrants depending on the particular situation, their comfort with specific subject areas, and their response to different people.

Specific conditions or situations also affect listening behavior. Physical factors like sitting in an uncomfortable chair, interacting in a room that is too hot or too cold, being in a noisy environment, or looking into bright light all affect listening. Listening is also negatively affected when listeners are uninterested in a speaker's views, disagree with what the speaker is saying, or have their mind made up and are therefore interested only in their own personal thoughts and ideas.

Motivation

It is important to acknowledge that we may never fully understand the actions of others. However, behavior is motivated (Garrett, 1982). It is important to recognize that the attainment of a client's goals depends in large part on the client's own motivation. In his book, *A Career in Speech Pathology,* Van Riper (1979) comments that "perhaps the most important of all the clinical skills required for effective therapy is the clinician's ability to motivate his [or her] clients" (p. 82). Van Riper shares several personal anecdotes from his career that illustrate the importance of motivation. One unusual but certainly illustrative story is retold here:

> One day a very determined young lady phoned and demanded an immediate appointment for herself and her husband. This is what she said: "We were married yesterday after a whirlwind courtship. I had never heard my husband stutter before but he's been stuttering horribly ever since the ceremony. I love him but I'm not going to bed with a monster until I'm sure that he can be helped. Can you cure him? We have separate rooms at the Burdick Hotel and must see you immediately. Can we come up right now?"
>
> Toujours l'amour, of course! The young man was indeed a very severe stutterer, gasping sequentially and compulsively until he blew himself up like a balloon, and only then could he utter the word he was trying to say. Pretty monosymptomatic, too. I told his wife, who did all the talking, that I didn't know if I could help him but I'd try. She turned to her man and laid it on the line. "OK, we'll see. I'll give you three weeks before I go after an annulment. Meanwhile, you'll sleep alone." A pretty hard-nosed gal. Well, I've never had any stutterer work harder than that man, day and night. Self-therapy at its best. All I had to do was make a suggestion, explain a procedure or point out a goal. He improved very quickly and soon eliminated all the gasping. Nevertheless, I was highly conscious of the calendar. Just before the three weeks were up, the man came in with a big cat-that-ate-the-canary grin on his face. "Well, Doc," he said, "I'm married at last, thanks to you." (pp. 94-95)

Motivation is enhanced when clinicians and clients have the same goals. Both parties also benefit when everyone is aware of the purposes of an interaction, how any information shared will be used, and what is expected of the participants. Some basic principles that affect motivation include the following:

1. Motivation will be high if a goal to be achieved is important to the person and there is a good possibility of reaching that goal.

2. Motivation will be facilitated, even when the client's motives differ from those of the clinician, if the client can identify with and relate to the clinician.

3. Many goals or achievements have a primary value to one person (e.g., the clinician), but only an incidental value to another person (e.g., the interviewee). In this case, one of the clinician's primary aims will be to link what is deemed important to accomplish to something that is of greater concern or value to the client.

4. Motivation is often facilitated if one does enough learning about something to generate at least a moderate level of anxiety about it.

5. Motivation is enhanced if a clinician is concerned more about the ongoing implementation of the process than about the goals alone.

6. Motivation is often increased when there is shared effort and responsibility. If the establishment of goals is desired, involving the party being interviewed or counseled in the decision-making process will typically facilitate motivation. However, there are exceptions to this—some individuals from linguistically and culturally diverse backgrounds who come from more authoritarian (rather than more democratic) cultures will expect that specific advice, suggestions, and directions come from the interviewer or counselor.

7. If some type of exchange of information or the acquisition of a skill is desired, then in general the flow of influence between the parties should be reciprocal. Motivated learning is sustained best by a reciprocal flow of information and influence.

8. Motivation is affected by the frequency of contact between the parties, by tasks that are perceived as being unfinished, by rewards that are acquired on an unpredictable schedule, and by information that is received in appropriate increments.

9. Success bequeaths success! Success with incremental small steps along the way facilitates long-range success toward larger overall goals.

These factors, although by no means all-inclusive, do provide a number of variables that relate to motivation in interviewing, counseling, and other clinical activities.

Rapport

No interviewer or counselor will get very far without establishing rapport with clients (Ivey, 1994). Establishing rapport is a process of creating and maintaining trust, confidence, and goodwill between the parties. The development and maintenance of rapport occur throughout interviewing or counseling sessions. The development of rapport is a process, not an event or something that is done or occurs at some particular time. It should be of concern at all times during clinical interactions.

Acceptance and respect are key components in establishing rapport (Moursund, 1993; Peterson & Marquardt, 1994). Through acceptance of the client, the clinician demonstrates respect. This respect, however, may not always be reciprocated. During an initial contact, indeed throughout the helping process, clinicians need to continually earn the respect and confidence of their clients and families. A specific procedure or even a series of procedures for establishing rapport cannot be offered. Rather, rapport is an ongoing process, a process initiated and maintained by our abilities to develop trusting, caring, accepting, and understanding relationships.

Benjamin (1981) suggests that there are three ways to achieve an understanding of another person:

1. Study information about a client, talk to others about the client, or listen as other people discuss the client. Hearing others talk about the client is clearly the most remote method of learning about the client, and often the most unreliable.

2. View a client through one's own eyes. Essentially, a clinician uses his or her internal frame of reference to view a client's background, experiences, feelings, and imagination.

3. Try to understand *with* the other person. In effect, clinicians try to understand a client by attempting to adopt the client's internal frame of reference in place of their own. Clinicians attempt to see how clients think, feel, and view the world. It can be very useful to strive to achieve this third level of understanding.

The development of rapport is ultimately influenced by the personalities of the individuals involved and by the professionals' abilities and skills. Thus, two clinicians using the same techniques or comments to facilitate respect and acceptance may not achieve the same results. However, being genuinely interested in people and giving clients direct, undivided attention are two excellent ways to start on the path to rapport.

There are, conversely, actions that have detrimental effects on the establishment of rapport. Showing too much "curiosity" or getting too personal hinders the development of rapport. Showing shock or surprise at something the other party says or does can also seriously undermine a relationship. Thus, taking in stride what may be said or done can help maintain a close, harmonious working relationship with others.

When clinicians notice that a relationship with a client is developing negatively, it is time to evaluate whether they are doing or saying something that is contributing to the problem. If there is no apparent cause or source of the negativity, one way for clinicians to gain or rebuild the interviewee's confidence and trust is to continue trying to understand the reasons for the difficulties. Clinicians can demonstrate consistent support and, if necessary, provide reassurance that they are not disapproving of their client's behavior.

In summary, rapport begins to develop before or during the first meeting and continues on throughout the course of the relationship. It encompasses the clinician's attempts to achieve cooperation and harmony with the client throughout their interactions together. In general, an honest and frank approach, in which interest in and sincerity toward the patient are demonstrated, will help establish a positive working relationship.

Concluding Comments

There are a number of prerequisites for effective interviewing. These include specific interviewer characteristics—spontaneity, flexibility, concentration, and specific facilitating conditions such as the presence of sensitivity and objectivity, good listening by both parties, motivation, and the development and maintenance of rapport. Each of these factors is important in the overall effectiveness of interviewing and counseling activities. Effective interactions do not occur accidentally. They are the result of refined clinical skills, empathy and clinical insight, cultural awareness and sensitivity, appropriate helping attitudes, and hard work.

Chapter *3*

Physical and Emotional Factors That Affect Communication

Chapter 2 included discussion of prerequisite interviewer characteristics and other basic factors that facilitate rapport, understanding, and good communication. This chapter examines a number of other factors that affect communication between interviewing and counseling parties. These factors include conditions within the physical environment and emotional, familial, religious, cultural, educational, and psychological factors related to the participants. Effective clinicians are aware of these factors and are prepared to understand and deal appropriately with them within interviewing and counseling situations.

Physical Environment

The physical setting in which a clinician works influences the overall effectiveness of an interview (Donaghy, 1990; Purkey & Schmidt, 1987; Reilly, 1988). The environment should ensure privacy, appear professional, and be comfortable. There should be adequate time allowed for an interviewing or counseling session, and the environment should engender the feeling that an interviewer's time is devoted to clients or caregivers. Attention should also be paid to the interview seating arrangements. The clinical environment in which such matters are neglected may affect clients in ways that hamper the clinician's effectiveness.

Privacy

Offering privacy and being attentive to those who are served are critical in interviewing and counseling (Donaghy, 1990; Rae, 1988; Shertzer & Stone, 1980). Disruptions should be avoided because they detract from privacy, take time, and divert focus from the client. For example, clinicians should not take phone calls during a session if at all possible (Benjamin, 1981; Samovar & Hellweg, 1982; Taylor, 1992). Many professionals instruct their fellow workers to prevent interruptions and to hold all telephone calls during patient contacts. Such procedures help ensure the concentration and continuity necessary for a clinician to accomplish what needs to be done and for clients to feel that the clinician's time is truly devoted to them.

Disruptions often engender uncomfortable and unproductive feelings of awkwardness for clinicians as well as for their clients. When a clinician interrupts a session to conduct other forms of business—either in person or by telephone—clients may begin to feel that they are in the way, and such feelings can influence their future participation in any necessary activities. Meanwhile, the clinician may feel restricted about what can be said to the other party in the presence of the client, and therefore, the quality of the clinician's service suffers all around.

Privacy is also affected by the physical structure and appearance of the interview environment. A number of clinicians working with communicative disorders do not have private offices or workplaces that have been specifically designed for comfort, confidentiality, and privacy. For ethical and practical reasons, it is important that any deficiencies be corrected, or at least improved. Clinicians need secure facilities where privacy can be ensured and confidentiality maintained. Public discussion of private matters is inappropriate and unethical. The need for confidentiality also applies for written material—case files, test results, notes pertaining to clients—and the clinician's facilities should ensure privacy adequate for the safe handling of these items.

Appearance of the Setting

Moursund (1985) comments that a client's real introduction to a clinician begins not through words but through the client's visual impressions of the setting. The location, the furniture, the color scheme, the pictures on the wall, the activity levels, the sounds, even the smells, all influence a client's impressions of and feelings about a setting. First impressions affect how a client thinks not only about the facility but about the services rendered there and the capabilities of the clinician who works there. Thus, the client's first impression of the setting, whether or not it reflects accurately on the clinician, can influence how the clinician and the other party interact and relate to each other.

The facilities in which professional services are provided should be clean, well lighted, as comfortable as possible, and free from distractions (Martin, 1994; Tomblin, 1994). The facilities should appear professional. Even in the worst possible place, there is something that can be done to make the environment look like someone cares enough to try to provide a pleasant atmosphere. A few decorations like plants and pictures, as well as the use of soft colors, can brighten up almost any environment. It is good to remember these comments from McCroskey, Richmond, and Stewart (1986):

> *Research indicates that when placed in any ugly room, people become discontented, irritable, bored, fatigued, and generally want out of the environment. Conversely, people placed in attractive surroundings work harder, are less fatigued, communicate more, are less irritable, and do not mind remaining in the setting for a reasonable period of time.* (p. 135)

Time

The time that is available and the way that time is handled affect interviewing and counseling efforts (McCroskey et al., 1986; Samovar & Hellweg, 1982). It is important not merely to have adequate time but also to appear to have adequate time. The appearance of adequate time is particularly important with some individuals from diverse ethnic groups. For example, within the Hispanic culture, at least a brief period of informal, friendly conversation sets the stage for subsequent discussions to occur. "Getting down to business" immediately or appearing hurried may be considered rude to many Hispanics (Anderson & Fenichel, 1989; Zuniga, 1992). Also, some native Americans will not discuss areas of personal concern if they feel rushed or hurried (Anderson & Fenichel, 1989; Roseberry-McKibbin, 1995).

The actual length of an interaction will vary according to the setting, the purposes of a meeting, and the individuals involved. Prior to any meeting, the interviewee should be provided with a general indication of the amount of time that will be involved. This general indication can be given when an appointment is made or at the beginning of the interview, or preferably on both occasions. A participant who is aware of the time that will be involved can make any necessary arrangements for such time and will come into an interview with clear expectations regarding the clinician's time.

Interviews that last longer than 45 to 60 minutes are typically exhausting and usually become nonproductive (Donaghy, 1990; Enelow & Swisher, 1986; Garrett, 1982). In cases where interviews are expected to last longer, it may be useful to take a break or to continue the discussion on another occasion. If either party experiences fatigue, an interaction should be discontinued. Another meeting can then be scheduled to complete any unfinished business (Benjamin, 1981; Kozloff, 1994).

The impression of having adequate time for the client is conveyed by the clinician's actions and words, as mentioned before, and even by the physical setting itself. A relatively clean work area conveys the impression that the clinician is organized and that time is to be devoted specifically to the client. Having any test materials, files, or other needed items available and handy expedites services, reduces any impressions of disorganization, and minimizes the need for unnecessary delays or interruptions during the session.

One important aspect of time management is promptness (Dillard & Reilly, 1988b; Meier & Davis, 1993). Being prompt is particularly valued by people from Anglo-European backgrounds. From this Anglo-European perspective, when one party to an interview is late, the other party often begins to develop negative feelings. Clinicians who are late for a meeting typically encounter clients who have already developed some agitation. Of course, the later any clinician is, the greater the agitation. Clinicians who consistently run late do themselves and their clients a disservice, and probably need to examine their ability to manage time. However, the value of time use and promptness is not seen across all cultures. Thus, clinicians who work with individuals from certain cultural backgrounds where adherence to time is less important may need to clearly communicate the need for promptness, and why it is considered important to them and their schedule.

Seating Arrangements and Distance

The physical seating arrangements and distance between the parties has received attention in the literature of interviewing and counseling (Benjamin, 1981; Donaghy, 1990; Edinburg, Zinberg, & Kelman, 1975; Knapp & Hall, 1992; McCroskey et al., 1986; Stewart & Cash, 1994). These arrangements, as well as the more obvious physical considerations, such as providing comfortable, appropriately sized chairs for the participants and minimizing any visual and auditory distractions, deserve the clinician's attention.

There is no absolute agreement among clinicians or researchers concerning which particular seating arrangement results in optimal communication. Years ago, Riley (1972) studied the effects of seating arrangements during counseling interviews and found that, although spatial arrangements did influence the clients' perceptions of the counseling relationship, no one specific arrangement emerged as being consistently superior. Rather, Riley found that clinicians' abilities, their actual behavior during interactions, and the relationships created between the parties were more important than the location of the seats. This does not mean, however, that the physical arrangements of the interview should not be considered.

One of the most comfortable and productive seating arrangements occurs when the parties sit somewhat close together at a 90-degree angle to each other with a small table between them (Benjamin, 1981; Taylor, 1992). This arrangement allows either participant to look directly at the other person, or to look straight ahead without appearing to wish to avoid eye contact. It is then simple and natural to look away to ponder information or determine what to say next. The use of a small table introduces an unobtrusive object that can mitigate any threat or discomfort that could result from there being open space between the participants. Such arrangements have considerable merit but may not always be possible and are probably not the most critical factor in any interaction. It is, however, important for an interpreter, if one is needed, to be within view of all participants.

The distance that separates participants during interactions has been discussed by a number of authorities (e.g., Cormier & Hackney, 1987; Hall, 1964; Mehrabian, 1972; Smith, 1973; Stewart & Cash, 1994). It is well accepted that smaller distances between people convey feelings of closer and more intimate communication. Greater distances are perceived as accompanying greater formality and less intimate communication (Mehrabian, 1968). All individuals have specific spatial expectations, and to avoid the disruption of communication, clinicians should strive to determine and respect these expectations (Hall, 1964). Generally, a distance of about three feet, or an arm's length, is appropriate (Stewart & Cash, 1994). Less space or extreme distance can inhibit effective communication (Cormier & Hackney, 1987; Roberts & Bouchard, 1989). An ideal distance is often related to participants' genders, ages, and cultural backgrounds (see Burgoon, 1994; Kleinke, 1986; McCroskey et al., 1986; Roseberry-McKibbin, 1995).

The following are some general observations concerning distance:

- Women tend to use less distance than men.
- Somewhere around 4 to 8 years of age, children adopt adult space norms. Prior to that time, spatial requirements may vary considerably among children.
- People who know each other, who have in effect already established a relationship, utilize less space than people who are beginning a relationship. Similarly, less distance is typically seen when participants relate well with each other.
- Distances are related in general to culture. For example, people of Hispanic, Italian, Latin American, Jewish, Middle Eastern, and Puerto Rican heritages tend to employ shorter distances between parties when talking. Conversely, persons of European/American, Chinese, German, and Japanese backgrounds tend to be more comfortable communicating from greater distances (see Abdrabbah, 1984; Irujo, 1988; Long, 1992; Roseberry-McKibbin, 1995; Sharifzadeh, 1992).
- People possessing a large degree of status and authority tend to feel comfortable relating from less distance; people with less status and authority tend to desire greater distance.

Again, these are general observations only; there are many individual exceptions. Interviewers and counselors want to position themselves as close to their patients as is comfortable and otherwise appropriate. They also need to make judgments about seating arrangements, with a view toward promoting optimal communication while minimizing discomfort in the other party.

Attitudes and Background Factors

In addition to the various environmental factors that influence interviews, the participants' attitudes also must be considered. An *attitude* may be thought of as a mental position; a feeling; or emotion toward a fact, a state, a situation, another person, or a group of people. Attitudes are influenced by cultural background and heritage, educational background, and previous life experiences. They are expressed in behavior, manners, beliefs, and values. Attitudes influence perceptions, and, thus, communication.

Clinicians must accept the reality of never being able to comprehend all the factors behind a client's attitudes. It is important simply to recognize that some individuals will have negative attitudes like prejudice, anger, and resentment, for whatever reasons. The clinician may need to accept their presence without developing negative feelings toward the other person. Acceptance involves a positive and active understanding of the client's feelings; but, interviewers do not have to condone and should not reinforce unacceptable attitudes or behaviors (Garrett, 1982).

According to Rich (1968), communication in interviews is affected by a number of variables such as age, intelligence, cultural background, previous contacts and relationships with the clinician or the setting, the presence of specific difficulties (e.g., a language barrier or an emotional disturbance), and whether an interaction is the first meeting or part of a series of interactions between the participants. Also influential are educational background, family, friends, language abilities, religious background and beliefs, socioeconomic status, even coming from a rural or urban environment. In the following sections, several of these factors are introduced and some brief comments are made; however, it is beyond the scope of this book to describe them in great detail. The conscientious clinician will realize that careful analysis of these variables may be necessary on a case-by-case basis.

Support from Family and Friends

The support or lack of support that clients receive from their friends and families can affect the provision of services. Clinicians often seek the help of family members to complete case histories, to assist directly in remediative efforts, and to help promote the generalization of newly established communicative skills—that is, to encourage the use of new skills in a variety of situations. Among many cultures, special or rehabilitative services are a "family affair"; it is a mistake to treat the individual in isolation. For example, in the Carolinian and Chamorro cultures of Micronesia, major decisions are not finalized until older family members agree (Hammer, 1994).

In some settings, a client's friends or other acquaintances may be involved in clinical efforts by providing transportation to the clinic or educational setting, providing information about a client, or assisting with specific treatment activities. At other times, someone like a client's co-worker, employer, or teacher may be at least indirectly involved by helping to adjust the client's schedule so the individual can be seen for services. Support and encouragement for these efforts of others is important. Without such help, services for the individual may not be possible.

Clients may receive moral support and encouragement, in varying degrees, from their families, friends, or caregivers. The presence and quality of this support can influence what happens in the clinical setting. For example, a child who is teased by peers about being enrolled for therapeutic help may be reluctant to cooperate fully with the clinician. In general, work with clients is positively affected when family and friends support the clinician's efforts. Conversely, a clinician's efforts are negatively affected when family or friends withhold support; for example, when they refuse to acknowledge that a problem exists or do not believe help is necessary. It is, therefore, important for clinicians to be aware of the type and level of support patients are receiving from family and friends. In some instances, this will be the basis for understanding certain unproductive attitudes and for beginning a process of modifying certain feelings.

Cultural Heritage

Cultural heritage is an extremely powerful variable in people's lives, holding paramount importance for individuals and having a deep influence on thoughts, attitudes, and actions. The effects of cultural heritage operate at both conscious and unconscious levels within all individuals. As Pederson and Ivey (1993), both of whom have written extensively in areas of multicultural communication, interviewing, and counseling, note:

> *Culture controls our lives. We may attend to our culturally learned assumptions or we may ignore them, but in either case, these assumptions will continue to shape our decisions. Culture is not something outside ourselves, but, rather, an internalized perspective that combines the teaching of every significant person or group we have experienced, read about, or heard about and from whom we have learned something. . . . (p. 1)*

Certainly no culture is inherently better or worse than another, but we tend to judge individuals from other cultures in light of our own cultural patterns and values. To work effectively with people from diverse cultures, clinicians need a strong grounding in cultural relativity. Clinicians can begin moving toward more effective understanding and interactions as they gain greater knowledge about their clients' cultures, as they learn, for example, how the various mores of a culture are likely to influence attitudes and behavior. However, even if professionals do not have a full understanding or appreciation of the cultures they encounter, they are still obligated to respect their clients and any cultural differences that may be present. Several valuable resources for learning more about culture and working with different cultural groups include Battle (1993a), Lynch and Hanson (1992a), Paniagua (1994), Pederson (1985), Pederson, Draguns, Lonner, and Trimble (1989), Pederson and Ivey (1993), and Roseberry-McKibbin (1995).

Religious Beliefs

Clinical work is sometimes affected by a client's religious convictions. Some years ago, McDonald (1962) cited an example of a child with a severe communication impairment whose family refused to accept clinical service because the notion of therapeutic intervention violated their religious beliefs. Taoism, for example, is practiced by many Chinese people. As Ima and Cheng (1989) note:

> *Taoism promotes passivity, and those that practice it may display a sense of fatalism about events surrounding them, resulting in resignation and inaction. This basic principle of nonintervention may have a deleterious effect when parents are asked to approve interventions for remediation of language or learning disorders.* (pp. 7-8)

A different example of the influence of religious beliefs, and ill feelings that can occur, may be seen when a clinician fails to recognize distinctive holidays, celebrations, days of worship, or religious terminology. Is the clinician, for example, to speak of the church, the temple, the synagogue, or the mosque?

Another effect of religious belief is illustrated by the former patient of one of my colleagues. A very religious young man, in his early twenties, enrolled for clinical treatment to remedy a /w/ for /r/ which was causing him considerable embarrassment. Through intensive clinical treatment, the /r/ was developed; however, it was this patient's belief that the sound had developed because of his intensive prayer rather than because of the services rendered—God had made the difference, not the therapist. My colleague still feels that her services also had something to do with this client's improvement.

Clinicians need to recognize the central importance religious beliefs hold for many people, and that clients' attitudes toward a variety of subjects may be influenced by them. In some cases, the support or lack of support of fellow church members can affect some clients' attitudes toward services offered. Clinicians should be attuned to detect the presence of such influences and be prepared to deal with them, if needed.

Education and Language Use

Education is another factor that influences communication in interview situations. A client's education may have come from formal schooling, real-world experience, or sometimes both. Typically, interviewers and counselors have to adjust to wide ranges in the kind and degree of knowledge possessed by clients.

It can be helpful for clinicians to remind themselves of the amount and type of education they themselves have experienced. Most professionals working with communicative disorders have completed at least 18 or 19 years of formal education, the last several of which have included intensive graduate-level academic coursework and clinical experience with communicative development and disorders. Few interviewees will have such an educational base. What is very familiar to the clinician frequently is new territory to others.

In general, clients' levels of knowledge are influenced by what they have experienced in life, not by the diplomas or degrees they may hold. The knowledge of a person with a doctoral degree in advanced physics may differ dramatically from the knowledge of a person with a doctoral degree in child development. But a person with little formal schooling may know considerably more about children and the development of communication than someone who holds several college degrees. Clinicians need to look beyond the specific number of years of education to assess an interviewee's knowledge about subjects of discussion.

The words clinicians use and the details of descriptions should correspond to the level of knowledge possessed by the client. In general, the longer clients have been exposed to treatment situations, the more familiarity they sometimes have with the type of information a clinician has to present. Faulty communication not only causes confusion and misunderstanding in the present, it can affect future interactions if clients begin to develop negative feelings toward the clinician. Words can be a clinician's best allies—or they can make the clinician appear condescending, insensitive, uncommunicative, uncaring, even pompous or arrogant (Enelow & Swisher, 1986).

One problem for an interviewer or counselor in any professional field is the use of technical jargon. As Chapter 6 describes in more detail, there is a considerable amount of technical jargon in communicative disorders. This terminology is useful for communicating with others working in the field or in related professions, but its use can be counterproductive for communicating with most nonprofessionals. Of course, clinicians can adjust the use of technical terminology according to the client's clinical experience. The patient involved in ongoing clinical treatment may understand terms like "articulation," "final consonant deletion," "conductive hearing loss," or "impedance," but it is unlikely that new patients will understand such terms.

One dictionary defines *jargon* as noncoherent gibberish; the use of professional jargon can be just that to many people. McFarlane, Fujiki, and Brinton (1984) provide an excellent example of how clients can interpret the use of specific jargon in communicative disorders. They comment that "to most people a *TACL* is a football maneuver, an *Arizona* is a state and a *PPVT* sounds like a childhood obscenity" (p. 9). Clinicians need to be careful in their use of acronyms, labels, and specialized terms. "Using direct, easily understood language may be the most basic step in maintaining an atmosphere that will allow all parties to make contributions, ask questions, and discuss the child's [or adult's] problem" (McFarlane et al., 1984, p. 10).

Age

Many young clinicians fear not being accepted or not being perceived as credible because of their age. A clinician's age can be a factor in some interactions, particularly with some members of linguistically and culturally diverse groups where age is more respected or revered than in the general U.S. culture. For example, in the Muslim culture, according to Nellum-Davis, "elders are considered authorities. Older clients will not comply when younger clinicians give them instructions or use direct requests using imperatives. Indirect requests and suggestions are the desired methods" (1993, p. 310). It is also particularly important for younger clinicians to use family names or titles, rather than first names, with many older clients.

In general, working with older persons is different than working with younger people. In their book, *Interviewing and Patient Care*, Enelow and Swisher (1986) devote an entire chapter to interviewing older adults. This chapter is highly recommended to students and professionals in all areas of health care. The following paragraphs paraphrase part of their work.

• Illness is much more common in the elderly, although it should not necessarily be accepted as the norm. The elderly often have multiple chronic medical problems. Because of the prevalence of multiple problems, which are sometimes accompanied by denial, effective interviewing and the accurate taking of case histories play a crucial role in the care of the elderly.

• Remember that elderly clients grew up in a very different age. They have experienced world wars, depressions, the emergence of rapid communication and transportation systems, as well as the death of many close friends and family members. They may be survivors who have been on their own for many years and are sometimes fiercely independent. This attitude can sometimes make their care difficult.

Although older persons grew up in a different era, they are also products of the here and now. They watch television, read advertisements, and may talk to friends about miracle cures, miracle hearing aids, and so forth. They are also subject to the myths of today's youth-oriented society, to the notion, for example, that youth is beautiful and age unattractive. Their being thus grounded in two different eras can make interviewing older patients especially interesting.

• The physical setting can be critical when interviewing or counseling many older people. Adequate lighting is particularly important because many older patients have reduced aural and/or visual acuity. Light should clearly illuminate the interviewer's face to facilitate speechreading. Because many elderly persons do have decreased aural acuity, it is especially important to speak distinctly and with sufficient loudness.

• It is important to begin sessions with older clients by first introducing yourself. Older people were raised in a time when propriety and decorum were held in great respect, and politeness and courteousness help to set them at ease. Many older people prefer to be addressed by their surnames rather than their first names.

• Some older patients have difficulty responding to questions that pertain to their feelings or to psychological issues. Many older patients were raised in a social climate in which personal problems were not discussed openly—sometimes not even within one's own family. They may be hesitant to open up early in an interview; rather, they may wait until they feel a measure of trust in the clinician.

• The time it takes one to respond when asked a question or asked to perform certain tasks can increase with age. Many older patients are less likely to take risks and are less willing to make errors than younger patients. Hence, many older clients may ponder or cogitate longer before answering questions.

• Many older people depend on other family members for some type or degree of support. The clinician should consider whether another family member should also be interviewed when seeing the older patient. If there are indications of memory problems, it is particularly important to corroborate the information presented by the patient. (Adapted from Enelow & Swisher, 1986, pp. 148-153.)

There are thus a number of factors for clinicians to consider when dealing with older clients. Cohen and Speken (1985) warn that, with many older adults, it is particularly important to watch for signs of fatigue. Sometimes a series of several short interviews is considerably more productive than one long interview. These considerations are especially relevant when an older adult is in less than full health.

Before leaving this area, it is important to stress that the preceding comments about people who are older are generalizations that, where tendencies and patterns may be seen within the group, do not necessarily apply to all individuals from that group. *Ageism*—imposing our beliefs and values on what older persons can or cannot do, or should or should not do—must be avoided. Clinicians also need to avoid discrimination on the basis of age. Discrimination can be reflected in feelings that older people cannot really be helped or by avoiding them (Okun, 1992).

Age also can be a consideration in communication when the client is a younger person, particularly when a client is an adolescent and the clinician is considerably older. Haynes, Pindzola, and Emerick (1992) suggest a number of considerations for minimizing potential age discrepancy problems with adolescents. The following paragraphs are based on their work and the information is applicable to interviewers and counselors.

• Acquire an understanding of the many pressures and changes the teenager is experiencing: rapid physical growth, sexual maturation, conflicts between dependence and independence, a search for identity and life work, and intense group loyalty and identification. The empathy that flows from an understanding of these factors can be a powerful force in establishing a positive working relationship with adolescents.

• Understand that adolescents often have very intense desires to be like their peers. Thus, a number of adolescents may find it extremely difficult to reveal a communicative problem, even if they want help, since the problem may suggest frailty or difference. The adolescent may try to cover up the problem with a dense "it doesn't bother me" shell. Denial is often seen, but you cannot simply dismiss the individual with a shrug. A straightforward approach is recommended: acknowledge the forces that are influencing the individual, objectively point out the paths others have taken, and provide information about the economic and social penalties that can accrue from a communicative impairment. Basically, try to demonstrate by your demeanor and words that you care and can help.

• Do not try to act like a teenager. Empathy is not the same as identification; do not abandon your professional role for that of a teenager. Attempting to do so will weaken your effectiveness, look ludicrous, and invite rejection.

• Approach the adolescent with tolerance and good humor. Do not be shocked or annoyed by overstatements and superlatives. Sometimes teenagers will, in order to uphold their protective armor, resort to all sorts of strategies to confuse, defeat, or even anger the clinician. The ability to laugh at yourself and to use humor in a gentle manner can be a real asset.

• Demonstrate your competence to deal with the person and the problem at hand. At appropriate times, explain what you are doing, why you are using specific tests, how you will use any information you gain, and what therapy will involve. Approach the adolescent as an adult, not as a child. (Adapted from Haynes et al., 1992, pp. 19–20.)

Interviewing children can be a little difficult for some interviewers, particularly if they have not been around a lot of youngsters. As Shipley and Wood (1996) notes, it is helpful to recognize the following:

• Most children are used to talking with adults even if it is only with their caregivers, family members, babysitters, or teachers.

• Children respect and respond to being treated with courtesy and respect. Most youngsters like to be treated as "conversational equals."

• Like adults, children need a "comfort zone" of space. We do not want to violate their space by getting too close, at least initially. Conversely, we do not want to "put off" someone whose space comfort zone is less than ours by reacting to too much closeness. Also, be aware that many children are uncomfortable being touched by strangers or those with whom they have had little previous contact.

• Although children's vocabularies are still developing, they still know a lot about their language and world. If we listen and use vocabularies appropriate to their age, some 2- and 3-year olds can carry out very "adult" conversations.

• Children will generally talk openly with adults who listen, suggest topics for discussion, let the child take the lead, and do not act in a judgmental manner. However, some children from linguistically or culturally diverse backgrounds (e.g., those from Asian and native American groups) may have been trained to be silent and respectful in the presence of unfamiliar adults. Such children will need to get to know the adult before really opening up.

• Children will also talk rather openly if they trust the adult. Violate this trust and you may have a very nontalkative child. (Adapted from p. 26)

In summary, age can be a factor that influences interactions. The effects of age differences are minimized, however, when clinicians are sensitive to others and to various needs at different age levels, are more concerned with matters at hand than age differences, are self-confident, and are focused on providing the most effective services possible. Chapter 8 contains additional comments about age as it applies to cross-cultural practice.

Gender

There can be differences in interviewees' responses that are based on whether the clinician is male or female (Burgoon, 1994; Casciani, 1978; Giles & Street, 1994; Kleinke, 1986; McCroskey et al., 1986). Both clinicians and clients are subject to being influenced by the gender of the other party in the interview. A clinician's gender may affect his or her approach to a client, particularly a member of the opposite gender, as well as the way certain questions are worded. Similarly, some interviewees may feel free to respond to certain questions posed by a member of one gender, but feel quite hesitant to respond to the same questions when asked by a member of the opposite gender.

In verbal communication, females tend to disclose more information about themselves (or about their family and friends) and generally are more open, outgoing, and expressive. Males tend to be more reserved and less verbal (Burgoon, 1994; McCroskey et al., 1986). Women also tend to be less direct than men (Tannen, 1994). Regarding nonverbal behavior, females tend to exchange more eye contact and exhibit more facial emotion than males. Females also tend to smile more. Males are less likely to cry during interviews, but are more likely to show their anger through facial expressions (McCroskey et al., 1986).

Although the two genders exhibit different frequencies of communication behaviors, this does not mean that either sex is particularly more effective in delivering services. For example, Shertzer and Stone (1980) reviewed a series of studies regarding the role of gender in counselor effectiveness. They concluded that overall effectiveness as a counselor was unrelated to a clinician's gender.

As discussed in greater detail in Chapter 8, there are differences across cultures with regard to gender. For example, some Middle Eastern males might not want to be questioned by a female interviewer or they might not allow their wives to speak alone with an interviewer. Some Middle Eastern men, particularly those from traditional Muslim families, may view themselves as the "sole agents" of communication between the family and the clinician (Sharifzadeh, 1992).

Personality, Appearance, Attraction, and Prestige

Several other factors that can influence interviewing or counseling sessions include the participants' personalities and appearance, their attraction to each other, and their prestige (Cormier & Hackney, 1987; Goldstein & Higginbotham, 1991; Kleinke, 1986; Meier, 1989; Moursund, 1993; Samovar & Hellweg, 1982). The participants' personalities affect their ability and willingness to participate openly in an interview, particularly during initial sessions. Someone who is attracted to the other participant typically is more willing to communicate freely in an interview.

The clinician's appearance can influence a client's feelings and, subsequently, the course of an interview. Most authorities recommend that interviewers and counselors dress conservatively to convey a professional manner. Meier and Davis (1993) suggest that a counselor's attire becomes a problem when it calls attention to itself. Kleinke (1986) notes that people prefer professionals to dress formally enough to maintain an image of expertise but not so formally as to appear stuffy or inapproachable. Kleinke also notes that interviewers come across as more competent when their clothing is in style rather than out of date.

An interview encounter can be influenced by the "prestige" of the interviewer or the interviewee. For example, interviewees often approach an interaction with confidence and high expectations when the interviewer is a respected authority. Such pre-interview confidence may not be seen in the absence of such prestige. Likewise, a client's prestige within a community can influence some clinicians' delivery of services. The professional may approach—consciously or unconsciously—an encounter differently when clients or their families are well known or highly respected members of the community (i.e., public officials, prominent business people, sports figures, entertainers, physicians, or in well-known colleagues in the field of communicative disorders, or in education-related or allied health professions).

These observations are not meant to imply that clinicians should ever vary the quality of their service according to the prestige of their clients; however, it is important to recognize that different factors can influence clinical interactions. Variables like socioeconomic status, ethnicity, gender, appearance and attraction, and prestige should be understood as factors that can affect a clinician's behavior and attitudes. Such understanding helps interviewers recognize why certain feelings may be present.

Emotions

Feelings and emotional states affect clinicians and clients. Meier and Davis (1993) write that counselors look for the "big four" feelings—anger, sadness, fear, and joy. With clients, it is helpful to remember that these individuals or their loved ones are experiencing disabilities with respect to one of the most important human skills—the ability to communicate. It is natural, therefore, that a considerable amount of emotion often surrounds these impaired abilities.

The clinician should also recognize that many individuals react to stimuli on an emotional basis first, and then to actual content. The clinician may notice emotional responses within the client's verbal and nonverbal reactions to certain questions, statements, or comments. Such reactions may be obvious or quite subtle, and they can include relief, joy, surprise, shock, anger, or resentment. Positive emotional reactions are typically pleasurable for everyone involved, but ambivalent or negative reactions may be much more difficult to understand and deal with. We all experience a variety of complex emotions. Besides fear of the immediate situation and for the future, some of the more common emotions seen in interviewing and counseling situations are disappointment, guilt, anger, and anxiety.

Disappointment

Disappointment is a natural reaction when the reality of a situation does not correspond with someone's hopes or anticipations. We all experience this emotion when what we expect or hope for does not materialize. Clinicians can experience disappointment when information is not accepted in the way that they think it should be. Interviewees can experience disappointment when, for example, the presence of a particular disorder is confirmed, or when a poor prognosis is presented. Feelings of disappointment may be general in nature or they may be specific reactions to events. From whatever source, feelings of disappointment are natural human reactions. Clinicians need to be prepared to accept the fact that disappointment, as well as sadness, occurs and to help disappointed clients appreciate the reality and any positive aspects of their situations.

Guilt

The emotion of guilt is often closely related to the emotion of anxiety. Sometimes feelings of guilt are expressed during initial interview encounters. In other cases, feelings of guilt may not emerge until later on in a relationship. Sometimes clinicians begin to recognize these guilty feelings only as time passes and after repeated interactions with clients.

Guilt often occurs when parents feel they have "sinned," that they created a problem because of something they did, because they failed to do something as soon as possible, or because they did something that now appears to have been wrong (Hartbauer, 1978). Sometimes speech-language pathologists and audiologists actually engender these feelings in clients. Consider, for example, how some parents might react to certain commonly asked questions: Where else has your child been seen? Has your child seen a physician recently? What have you done to try to help? When did you first notice the problem? Other questions, which it may be necessary to have answers for, can also engender guilt: Did you use any alcohol or drugs during the pregnancy? Why did you discontinue therapy? Why did you...? Feelings of guilt or feelings of having been negligent can sometimes be intensified when clinicians suggest that early treatment would have been useful, that the problem could have been detected earlier, or that what was done for the client may not have been the most effective thing to do.

Clinicians may need to provide reassurance to counter feelings of guilt—by remaining objective, by listening to feelings of the client or the client's family members, by correcting any misperceptions they have or inaccurate information they may have received, and generally by helping these persons work through their guilty feelings. Guilt does not typically disappear after the first reassurance that "it is not your fault" or "it is OK." Rather, the reduction of guilty feelings takes time and sometimes requires gaining a more complete understanding of the situation. One of the major tasks of clinicians encountering clients with guilt is to help these individuals gain better perspectives on their situations so they can move forward with the tasks at hand.

It is inappropriate to provide false assurances in an attempt to modify feelings of guilt. There are times when clinicians cannot say, "It's OK." The task of clinicians in such instances is to help people move from counterproductive guilt to constructive feelings and activities—feelings and activities that will assist patients in the here and now and with the future. Involving people with guilt in certain treatment activities can be helpful for them because concern then becomes focused on the present (Zebrowski & Schum, 1993). Individuals experiencing guilt often benefit when they are made to feel part of the solution rather than part of the problem.

Guilt also can be related to cultural beliefs. For example, within some groups of the Filipino culture, there is a belief that a child with a handicapping condition is due to parents' or ancestors' sins (Chan, 1992a). Among some Middle Easterners, a mother may be held responsible and feel guilty if a child is born with a disability, while the father feels shame and a sense of personal defeat. Such feelings can be associated with denial, isolation, overprotection, or even abandonment of the child (Sharifzadeh, 1992). Among some Samoans, children are viewed as gifts from God; thus, a handicapped child can be interpreted as God's displeasure with the family (Mokuau & Tauili'ili, 1992).

Anger

Anger can have a number of sources. Hackney and Cormier (1994) write that

> *Different kinds of stimuli often elicit anger. One such stimulus is **frustration.** Others are **threat** and **fear.** Conditions such as competition, jealousy, and thwarted aspirations can become threats that elicit angry responses. Anger often represents negative feelings about oneself and/or others. Many times, fear is concealed by an outburst of anger. In such cases the anger becomes a defensive reaction because the person does not feel safe enough to express fear. Anger is also a cover-up for hurt. Beneath strong aggressive outbursts are often deep feelings of vulnerability and pain. . . . Remember that anger covers a broad group of feelings and can be expressed in many ways.* (p. 96)

Thus, the emotion of anger is often a mechanism employed, consciously or unconsciously, for self-protection. Hartbauer (1978) feels that expressions of anger may occur for several reasons: The client may not understand the situation, the alternatives, the need for treatment, or may be unhappy about being unable to resolve the problems being experienced.

When a client's anger is directed at clinicians, they need to consider what aspects of their own behavior may be creating or engendering the problem. Lateness, talking over the client's head, using language that is too technical, appearing insensitive, failing to truly understand what the client is saying—all these are among the possible sources or contributors to a client's anger. At other times, of course, anger that is directed toward clinicians actually has little to do with them. Rather, the clinician may simply be the most available person on whom to vent some feelings.

Finally, be aware that anger may not be demonstrated by some individuals from certain cultural groups, even when an individual may be quite angry. For example, many Asians will not express their anger out of respect for the other person (Chan, 1992b). Individuals from the

Chamorro and Carolinian cultures tend to avoid conflict and refrain from expressing anger, particularly when interacting with persons who have more perceived authority (Hammer, 1994). Clinicians need to exercise care in assuming that, just because someone is not expressing anger, such feelings are not present.

Anxiety

There are many sources of anxiety that can accompany a communicative difficulty. A client may feel anxious because of uncertainties about the present and future course of the communicative difficulties and about the social, vocational, or educational consequences. Other sources of anxiety may be the clinician's personality, the methods or attitudes conveyed by the clinician, questions about the outcome of the clinician's efforts, or doubts whether the clinician will be able to handle the client's problems (Hartbauer, 1978). Feelings of anxiety are often present during initial encounters because people are unsure exactly what to expect. As the discussion of orientations in Chapter 4 indicates, many of these feelings of anxiety during initial encounters can be reduced by the provision of appropriate presession information.

Clinicians should be able to detect many instances of anxiety. These feelings may be seen in clients' direct verbalizations or in their hesitancy, passivity, anger, or verbally aggressive behavior. Often the open expression of anxiety should be encouraged because it allows clinicians to deal with areas of concern and, if necessary, helps provide clients with more objective, accurate information or with appropriate assurances.

A number of clients from linguistically or culturally diverse backgrounds may have considerable anxiety coming into interview situations, particularly if there is a language barrier or if a large group of professionals is present. It is often wise to keep groups of professionals rather small. Also, in many instances, an interpreter from the culture being seen may be beneficial (Roseberry-McKibbin, 1995).

Defensive Reactions and Defense Mechanisms

We all need to defend ourselves, to maintain a sense of self-esteem while securing time to begin resolving problems that would otherwise be too overwhelming; therefore, some degree of defensive behavior is often merited and useful (Shipley & Wood, 1996). However, defensive behavior can have a negative effect if it is used excessively, or when it conceals problems that truly need attention and resolution. Defensive behavior also can preclude successful communication, understanding, and cooperation. People exhibit various degrees of defensive behavior. Obviously, interactions will be affected differently by mild defensiveness versus very adamant defensive reactions.

Defensive feelings can be engendered when clients feel misunder-stood, or if they become frustrated when conflicting opinions arise—concerning, for example, whether or not someone has a problem, or the frequency or type of treatment needed. Defensiveness can result in aggressive behavior, extreme passivity, chronic disagreement with others, self-perceptions of omniscience or omnipotence, and/or the tendency to intellectualize.

Sigmund Freud's works with ego protection led to the description of a number of specific defense mechanisms—for example, denial, intel-lectualization, reaction formation, suppression, repression, rationaliza-tion, displacement, and projection—people employ. Clinicians working with communicative disorders are apt to encounter such defense mecha-nisms (Hutchinson, 1979; McDonald, 1962; Rollin, 1987). It should be noted and stressed that such defense mechanisms are frequently, though not always, employed unconsciously. The following section describes reac-tion formation, suppression, repression, rationalization, displacement, and projection. Chapter 9 addresses denial and intellectualization. For additional information on defense mechanisms, refer to Anna Freud (1967) or any of a number of textbooks in psychology.

Reaction Formation

A reaction formation may occur within some individuals when the emotions they experience are so shocking or contrary to their actual thoughts that the new feelings are considered unacceptable and inap-propriate. In reaction formation, individuals develop attitudes that are opposite to their real feelings about a subject and then adhere only to these newly created, more positive and "acceptable" thoughts. The individual's external reactions and activities then do not directly reflect or express the person's true feelings. For example, the mother who has a very deep resentment toward her severely handicapped child may actually immerse herself in exuberant involvement with her child, with charity organizations dealing with the child's disorder, and so forth.

Reaction formation is also exhibited by some individuals who fight against all odds in the hope that their loved one will be the one-in-a-million who overcomes some difficulty. These examples illustrate how the activities subsequent to a reaction formation can be positive while the real questions about how the individual truly feels remain unre-solved. The positive appearance of the reaction formation masks the real problem that still exists. As Clark (1994b) notes:

> *Although reaction formation can affect management negatively, it*
> *can also have a positive influence. In avoiding the initial urge to*
> *deny the diagnosis, some parents may become strong advocates for*
> *services to the hearing impaired or may become hearing providers*
> *themselves (Mitchell, 1988). However, it is certainly within the*
> *audiologist's [or speech-language pathologist's] purview to help direct*

parents appropriately so that during this period other family re-sponsibilities do not fall along the wayside. (p. 34)

The severity of reaction formation can vary across individuals. And, although some positive activities may occur subsequent to a reaction formation, there is still an underlying problem that needs resolution—how the individual really feels about the "unacceptable" subject. Hutchinson (1979) points out that reaction formation is difficult for untrained persons to deal with, and that referral for professional counseling is often indicated for people exhibiting this defense mechanism.

Suppression

Suppression is somewhat similar to self-control. It is a reaction in which individuals keep their impulses, wishes, and desires under control and out-of-view of others. Their true feelings may be held inside and even denied publicly. In some instances, this can be counterproductive for the person as well as for the clinician's treatment efforts.

Clinicians need to understand that, in accordance with the customs of some cultures, individuals from certain backgrounds tend not to express personal or negative feelings as it would be considered rude or otherwise inappropriate to share their real feelings with someone "in authority." Thus, particularly with individuals from some linguistically and culturally diverse backgrounds, care is necessary before presuming that suppression is being exhibited.

Repression

Repression has been described as being one step beyond suppression (Clarke, 1968). Rather than controlling or suppressing feelings, the person actually represses and henceforth is unable to recognize them. For this reason, at a conscious level, a problem does not exist and there is, therefore, little or no reason for concern or action.

Repression presents exasperating treatment difficulties for clinicians working with communicative disorders. Take, for example, the severe stutterer who has repressed any recognition of the problem, or the parent who has repressed awareness (and thereby any possible acceptance) of a nonverbal five-year-old's communication problem, or a hearing-impaired person who insists that the hearing is "clear as a bell." After all, for the person who represses, the problem does not exist.

Rationalization

Rationalization involves a logical but untrue explanation of some attitude or behavior. It typically allows an individual to explain why some expectation has not occurred (Shipley & Wood, 1996). Rationalization helps an individual maintain a positive opinion of self while attempting to justify certain actions or failures. From time to time most people have used rationalizations to explain away certain shortcomings or failures. A problem emerges, however, with the frequent, excessive, or counterproductive use of rationalization.

A clinician may encounter rationalization as a form of resistance to treatment. The patient may have "been too busy" to see the physician for the medical clearance that would have allowed the clinician to dispense the hearing aid or to begin voice therapy. There also may be a more general tendency to rationalize about the history of a problem. Rather than getting caught up in rationalizations about what did not get done, clinicians should focus on the positive actions that need to be accomplished—that is, where we need to go from here.

Displacement

Displacement occurs when an individual transfers hostile feelings from the person or problem that caused them onto a "safe" person or object. When doors get slammed, when someone acts aggressively toward innocent family pets, when children throw blocks or books from the table, when adults pick fights with their spouses—these occurrences frequently are examples of displaced emotion. The persons or events that triggered the anger or hostility lie elsewhere.

Displacement satisfies an immediate need to vent anger in a safer manner than would be possible by confronting the actual source of irritation. Besides the fact that it allows the individual to avoid addressing the real source of the hostile feelings, displacement can end up causing new problems because it also creates scapegoats.

Projection

Projection involves a distortion of reality that goes beyond displacement. The individual who employs this defense mechanism shifts responsibility to someone else. Feelings or motives that really belong to the individual are attributed to another person. Projections can be used to transfer blame, to excuse failures, or to minimize personality problems or weaknesses.

A person does not need to do anything to become the target of a projection. A physician can be blamed for failing to prevent or identify a problem, when in reality the patient should have had a checkup earlier. A teacher can be faulted for being a "bad teacher who doesn't like me," when in reality the student did not study for the test. A speech-language pathologist can be condemned for "not knowing what she's doing," when in reality the patient resisted therapy. The audiologist can be blamed because the hearing aid does not restore normal hearing. The spouse or family member can be faulted—for whatever reason.

Incidentally, there may be truth in some of these complaints on certain occasions. However, clients who employ projection are distorting reality in attempting to relocate the blame for their own failures or frustrations.

Clinicians must realize that it is not uncommon for them to be targets of such projections (Hutchinson, 1979; Schum, 1986; Shipley & Wood, 1996). If good service has been rendered, a patient's complaints may relate more to the need for ego protection than to something the clinician may or may not have done.

Some Advice for Clinicians

Lon Emerick has contributed to a number of fine resources dealing with interviewing, diagnosis, stuttering, and the clinical process for students and professionals working with communicative disorders. A considerable portion of the information in this section has been adapted from materials found in several of Emerick's works (Emerick, 1969; Emerick & Hatten, 1979; Haynes et al., 1992).

Throughout the present text, the point is made that both parties in the interview affect an interaction. Emerick (1969) indicates that a clinician, particularly a beginning clinician, may bring certain feelings or attitudes into an encounter that can influence the behavior of both parties. He describes several "hang-ups" sometimes found with beginning clinicians. One is a fear of not being accepted by parents as a professional because of age. Another is the fear of encountering a defensive parent who will not accept what the beginning clinician is conveying. The clinician also may fear being questioned by parents. Needless to say, these fears apply to more than just working with parents.

Emerick (1969) also reminds us that many clinicians can be too judgmental when viewing parents' or other people's behaviors. Based on his thoughts regarding working with parents, it is useful to consider the following points:.

• Every person has his or her unique needs and concerns. Parents, caregivers, spouses, and other concerned persons are more than just vehicles for gaining information or help with clinical treatment.

• Family members—whether children, significant others, parents, or other relatives—can be difficult to cope with, and the presence of a communicative disorder can accentuate any problems that may already exist.

• All observations must be carefully interpreted. Clinicians should avoid overinterpreting or prematurely interpreting their observations or impressions.

• People typically want what is best for their children, parents, relatives, and friends. As the discussion in Chapter 5 points out, individuals who have done the wrong thing have often done so for the right reasons. The clinician should assess behavior not only in terms of what was done but also in terms of why.

• Actions speak louder than words. When clinicians can demonstrate that their efforts produce changes in their clients' communicative abilities, their credibility is enhanced and other people are more willing to cooperate with them. Nothing beats effectiveness for engendering greater cooperation. (Adapted from Emerick, 1969, p. 11.)

Concluding Comments

This chapter describes a number of factors that influence the quality of communication in interview situations. Some of these factors, such as the immediate physical environment, are controlled directly by the interviewer. Other factors have to do more with what clients bring to an interview. Any of these factors can influence a clinician's overall effectiveness in delivering services. It is important for the clinician to monitor the effects of these factors—to determine, for example, when clients' or caregivers' attitudes or feelings are counterproductive to communicative improvement—and to make appropriate adjustments or suggestions for change.

Clinicians will need to work directly with some emotion-related difficulties, particularly as they affect a communicative disorder and its treatment. With some of the defense mechanisms described in this chapter, and some other concerns discussed in Chapter 9, there will be times when clinicians need to make referrals to other professionals. The competent clinician is willing and able to make such referrals, when necessary. Guidelines and suggestions for making referrals are in Chapter 10.

Skills and Techniques for Interviewing and Counseling

Effective interviewers and counselors have many skills and techniques in their repertoire that affect communication. Among these tools are several distinct kinds of questions, specific verbal and nonverbal behaviors, and a number of other clinical techniques that facilitate communication. Skilled clinicians are conscious of these tools and have learned to employ them purposefully. This chapter describes a number of these tools. But, before beginning these discussions, a listing of general suggestions for promoting appropriate interactions is presented.

General Suggestions

Bingham, Moore, and Gustad (1959) recommend a number of basic guidelines for use in interviewing. Their suggestions, still valid, are adapted and many are commented on in the following section. The suggestions that follow are appropriate for all interviewers and counselors.

- Decide beforehand what needs to be accomplished. Clinicians should have a good idea what needs to be done and what types of information need to be obtained or shared. For beginning interviewers, it is helpful to make a brief list of the major areas to be discussed to use as a reference.

- Learn as much as possible about the interviewee. This can be done both before and during the interview. If a client is from a linguistically or culturally diverse background, learn about that culture.

- Make sure the client understands in advance when the appointment will involve an interview.

- Make clear the approximate amount of time allotted for any interviewing or counseling session. If a client comes from a culture with a more relaxed view of time, this should be considered. The element of time may need to be addressed beforehand.

- Allow sufficient time for any interaction. Adequate time is needed for any presession preparation, the interview itself, and the collection of thoughts and any necessary paperwork afterward. Interviewing and counseling sessions are less effective when conducted on tight, counting-the-minutes schedules, or when clinicians are running behind schedule. Also, allow extra time when an interpreter is part of any interaction.

- Provide a private setting that maintains confidentiality.

- Learn to understand the other person's point of view. It is helpful to consider how we would react to the questions asked or the information that needs to be presented.

- Develop understanding and empathy.

- Understand your own personality and your beliefs and prejudices about different people and subjects. Everyone has ideas and opinions that need to be understood so they do not inappropriately affect interactions with others.

- Establish a relationship where confidence and trust can develop.

- Establish an atmosphere that is as pleasant and relaxed as possible. It is difficult for anyone to communicate effectively in unpleasant or tense situations. Clinicians are responsible for helping clients and families feel at ease and for engendering their willingness to share information and concerns.

- Help interviewees feel free to talk, and interfere as little as possible. Remember, the more you are talking, the less the interviewee is talking.

- Listen carefully. As discussed in the section on listening in Chapter 2, good attending skills are critical to true understanding.

- Be aware of the effects of fatigue. Either interviewers or interviewees can feel the effects of fatigue, which considerably reduces communication. When fatigue occurs, the participants should take a break or schedule another conference. Either of these options is better than trying to plod through an interview or cutting an interaction short at the risk of miscommunicating, failing to learn certain information, or failing to provide certain information.

- Avoid wasting time dwelling on unimportant matters, and avoid working at too slow a pace. Many interviewees react negatively to either of these problems. However, do recall that certain clients, particularly some individuals from linguistically and culturally diverse backgrounds, will expect at least a brief period of informal chit-chat before "getting down to business" (Larson & McKinley, 1995; Zuniga, 1992).

- Maintain control of the interview. Cover the points that must be addressed; conversation should not be allowed to wander to irrelevant topics. This consumes time and, in some instances, causes interviewees to question whether clinicians really know what they are doing.

- Use interviews discriminately. There is no need for an interview if the information to be discussed can be effectively obtained or provided by another means. Often, concerns can be taken care of in other ways and everyone's time and trouble can be saved.

- Make sure the topics addressed in an interview are truly important and that the issues are understood by interviewees. Resentment can be a real problem when interviewees question why certain information is needed. Certain questions or areas of discussion may be perceived as being highly personal. The reasons these areas require discussion may need to be addressed.

- Use interviews to gain as well as confirm information. Information that has been provided on a case history or by someone else may need to be confirmed by observation or discussion.

- Use interviews to gain subjective as well as objective information. For example, interviewees' opinions, attitudes, and beliefs are likely to have important influences on certain areas of discussion, or overall interaction patterns.

- Know your field. Clients are seeking the clinician's help and will expect that person to know the answers to their concerns and questions. However, if there is something the clinician does not know, it is far better to say "I don't know" than to provide inaccurate information. It is even better to say, "I don't know, but I will find out." Of course, it is then important to honor this commitment.

- Ask questions that help gain any information needed. Questions that are difficult to follow rarely elicit the desired information. Use terms that interviewees have a reasonable chance of understanding. For example, ask parents for their impressions of a child's oral mobility or use of interrogatives and they may respond, "Huh?"

- Ask one question at a time. A question with several parts often causes confusion that results in important points going unaddressed. Multiple-part questions also are very difficult for interpreters, when these persons are part of an interaction.

- Give respondents adequate opportunities to answer the questions posed. Some clients need more time than others to respond. When planning an interview, allow ample time for each topic to be addressed.

- Let interviewees tell their stories. Clients and caregivers suffering or involved with communicative impairments often have feelings about the causes and effects of the problems. They often come prepared to share their frustrations about coping with the communicative difficulties, fears about what lies ahead, hopes for securing adequate diagnosis or treatment, disappointment when problems have not been outgrown or remediated, or other such fears and frustrations. For the sake of any interactions that follow, it is vital that interviewees have the opportunity to share such feelings. Interviewees' stories also can provide clinicians with valuable insight into attitudes that may affect treatment. Interviewers who do not provide such opportunities can be viewed, justifiably, as being insensitive and incomplete in their work.

- Keep the interaction focused on the matters at hand. Various techniques useful for focusing or refocusing discussion are presented later in this chapter.
- Avoid assuming a lecturing role. Interviewees should view clinicians as knowledgeable people who are capable of helping. They should not be made to feel that they are in a role of inferiority or subservience.
- Be straightforward and honest. Cleverness and deceit are rarely, if ever, effective in interviews. One characteristic of European-American culture is to be somewhat "upfront" or "blunt." However, certain individuals from other cultures (e.g., Filipino and Japanese) are used to less directness. Some care is needed in this area, as described in Chapter 8.
- Look for the full meaning of each answer. Skilled practitioners carefully consider the actual words interviewees use, possible meanings behind those words, and any accompanying nonverbal behaviors exhibited.
- Be alert for inconsistencies in interviewee responses and, when they occur, double-check the information in question. This double checking must be handled skillfully and in a neutral manner, not in an obtrusive or accusatory manner. Avoid something like, "Earlier you said _____ , and now you are saying _____. Which is it?"
- Realize that there is a difference between a fact and someone's interpretation of a fact. There are differences between observable facts, alleged facts, inferences drawn from facts, and even inferences that masquerade as facts. It is important to distinguish between these representations and to view each in its proper perspective.
- Check representations of fact against your own observations. For example, a patient's parents might state that their child does not seem concerned about a speech problem, but the clinician's direct observation of the child would suggest otherwise.
- Do not assume that agreement means validity. Several people, a whole family, or a whole other group, may agree about something—but, that does not necessarily mean it is correct!
- Assume the honesty of statements, but always be hesitant to conclude that everything is actually the way it is represented. For example, some clients may say certain things they think a clinician wants to hear out of respect for that person's authority. There is certainly no need to distrust people in general; but professional judgments must be made carefully and tentatively. (Adapted from Bingham et al., 1959, pp. 64-77.)

These are useful guidelines for interviewing and counseling efforts. Many of the points are described in greater detail in this chapter or elsewhere in the book.

Questions in an Interview

Asking questions is the primary method used to obtain information from interviewees, particularly in interviews aimed at obtaining information. The use of questions helps clinicians secure information needed, clarify patients' statements, explore various thoughts that have been expressed, motivate people to communicate freely, and direct the focus of conversations (Brammer, 1993; Garrett, 1982; Shipley & Wood, 1996). The wording and the sequencing of questions guide interviewees into specific areas for further discussion or greater understanding. There are a number of good reasons for asking questions; however, the appeasement of curiosity is not a valid reason (Garrett, 1982). It is, therefore, important for interviewers to understand their motives and reasons for asking questions. If an interviewer does not know why a particular question is being asked, it should not be asked. It is also important to know the limitations of questions. As Pederson and Ivey (1993) comment:

> *Questions are the most frequently used—and overused—tool of interviewers and counselors. Questions can be used to encourage or discourage talking. Usually the questions are asked by the interviewer and answered by the interviewee, putting the interviewer in control of the situation. Questions have a great deal to do with power. When counselors lose control in an interview, they sometimes ask a new question as the means of recapturing control. Question-asking skills increase a counselor's ability to collect specific information, redirect the interview, or encourage the interviewee to disclose general information.* (p. 131)

There is more to the art of information gathering and posing questions than it might appear at first glance. There are three major types of questions: open or closed, primary or secondary, and neutral or leading questions (Stewart & Cash, 1994). Questions are:

1. Open or closed depending on how they are asked and the level of response specificity required.
2. Primary or secondary depending on the order in which they are presented and the level of response specificity required.
3. Neutral or leading depending on whether they are framed in a way that potentially biases or influences an interviewee's response.

In addition to these three ways of distinguishing between questions, interviewers also distinguish between questions as do reporters—they may employ *who, what, when, where, how,* and *why* questions to elicit distinct kinds of information. Questions, such as *is* or *was, could,* or *would,* may also be seen.

Open and Closed Questions

Open questions. Open questions allow patients or caregivers to respond in a number of possible ways. A response with specific types or increments of information is not required. "What brought you here today?" or "What are some of your concerns?" are examples of open questions. This type of question encourages interviewees to respond with information of particular interest to them, rather than within specifically identified areas of inquiry contained within a question. Open questions require respondents to be actively involved in the interview process and to organize and structure their thoughts before responding. An interviewer controls the general subject area with open questions, but the range of possible responses rests with the interviewee; thus, the client provides much of the specific direction but within the general framework of the question.

Because the object is to draw a client out, care should be taken to frame open questions so they cannot be answered with a simple "yes" or "no" or with only a short response. Frequently the interviewer will begin an open question with a phrase like "Tell me about..." or "What are...?"; for example:

"Tell me about Felicia's speech."
"What are some of your concerns?"

These examples illustrate how the general frame of reference (Felicia's speech, your concerns) is provided by the interviewer. The interviewee, however, may respond in a number of possible directions (Felicia's sound errors, correctly produced sounds, intelligibility, frustrations about speech, communicating with others, effects on academics, parental frustrations, effects of treatment, and so on).

Another open-ended method of securing certain information is to repeat a respondent's key words:

CLIENT: I'm concerned about problems with the tongue.
CLINICIAN: The tongue?

CLIENT: I think my son may have a speech problem.
CLINICIAN: A speech problem? Tell me about it.

CLIENT: I think my hearing has gone downhill.
CLINICIAN: Downhill?

According to Stewart and Cash (1994), several advantages of open questions include:

- Encouraging the party being interviewed to talk
- Communicating interest in the other party
- Encouraging clients in a nonthreatening manner by providing more than one response option
- Learning the issues and concerns that patients feel are particularly important
- Allowing the other party to provide information that might otherwise not have occurred to the interviewer
- Helping reveal clients' knowledge or understanding about certain matters
- Revealing topics about which interviewees or counselees have feelings and questions

- Revealing respondents' frames of references, or even prejudices and stereo-
typed attitudes (Adapted from p. 64.)

A further advantage of open questions is that they tend to elicit responses that are more accurate and reliable than many responses to closed questions (Enelow & Swisher, 1986). Open questions are also useful in helping many individuals from linguistically and culturally diverse backgrounds express themselves more freely (Culatta & Goldberg, 1995).

Open questions, however, do have some disadvantages. For one thing, using them can be very time-consuming. They may elicit overly long and unorganized answers that may require a number of follow-up questions. Also, by using open questions respondents may end up address-
ing information and feelings that are not particularly pertinent, or they may fail to provide important information because they think it is incidental or unimportant, or they get sidetracked with another topic. An-
other potential disadvantage is that the use of open questions requires a considerable degree of skill. Inexperienced interviewers often find it difficult to control conversational directions with open questions (Shipley & Wood, 1996; Stewart & Cash, 1994). Despite these potential difficulties, though, skillfully asked open questions help interviewers gain important information and insight that is simply not possible when inter-
viewers rely too much on closed questions.

Closed questions.   Closed questions are much more highly structured than open questions—they focus or limit an interviewee's responses. They are typically used to obtain specific increments of information. These types of questions are particularly helpful when interviewers need to check their impressions against those of their interviewees (Nirenberg, 1968). There are three basic levels of closed questions: moderately closed questions, highly closed questions, and bipolar questions (Stewart & Cash, 1994). *Moderately closed questions* require clients to provide specific pieces of information; *highly closed questions* allow interviewees to choose among alternative answers; and *bipolar ques-
tions* offer only two response choices.

> *Moderately Closed Questions:* "Have you had ear infections?" "How many ear infections have you had?" "Have you ever considered speech therapy?" "How frequently does your child stutter?" "Would you like a referral for _____?"
>
> *Highly Closed Questions:* "Did you have one, two, or three ear infections last winter?" "Does your child stutter occasionally, frequently, or all the time?" "Would you like a morning, afternoon, or early evening appoint-
ment?"
>
> *Bipolar Questions:* "Do you have ear infections?" "Does your child stut-
ter?" "Did you do your homework?" "Did you contact the doctor?" "Would you like to schedule an appointment?"

Responses to these different types of closed questions differ. Among the three types of closed questions, moderately closed questions offer respondents the most response options, followed by highly closed questions. Responses to bipolar questions are the most restrictive, resulting in responses such as yes or no, like or dislike, approve or disapprove, agree or disagree, and so forth. Speech and hearing specialists can employ all three types of closed questions during an interview. Knowing that each question type produces a different type of response, interviewers vary their use of closed questions according to the type of information needed.

Closed questions have a number of advantages. They are relatively easy to control and thus easy for beginning interviewers to use. They tend to result in short answers that are relatively easy to analyze; thus, a large number of closed questions can be asked in a relatively short period of time. Further, closed questions are generally easy for interviewees to answer because they do not require detailed explanations (Stewart & Cash, 1994).

Relying on too many closed questions, however, can be detrimental to a relationship or can result in clinicians not understanding some of an interviewee's major areas of concern or interest. Hegde and Davis (1995) comment that it is not uncommon for beginning student clinicians to have difficulties establishing rapport during initial interviews, at least in part because of insufficient knowledge or experience knowing when and how to use closed questions. Clients who are interviewed primarily with closed questions can also feel that clinicians are performing a "robot-like" interview where a question is asked, the answer given, another question asked, this question is answered, and so forth.

Open and closed questions each have their own strengths and weaknesses and both are useful in interviewing. Open questions tend to produce longer responses that contain a good deal of general information, whereas closed questions tend to produce shorter responses containing specific pieces of information (Shipley & Wood, 1996). Both types of information are useful in working with communicative disorders, and a clinician's ability to employ both types of questions skillfully is important for effective interviewing.

Primary and Secondary Questions

Primary questions introduce new topics, or new areas within a topic. The introduction of a primary question does not require any preceding contextual cues. For example, an interviewer might ask, "Do you think your daughter might have a hearing loss?" When the interviewee responds to the primary question, the clinician may then need to follow up with one or more secondary questions to elicit more specific or detailed information. The interviewer might ask: "What leads you to feel that way?" "How long have you noticed this?" "Are there times she seems to be missing what you're saying?" and so forth. Thus, secondary questions are really follow-up questions that help elicit more detailed pieces of information.

Neutral and Leading Questions

Questions can be distinguished as neutral or leading, depending on whether they are framed in a way that could influence an interviewee's response (Donaghy, 1990). Neutral questions are unbiased, allowing respondents to choose their answers without being unduly influenced by the interviewer. Questions such as "How do you feel about _____?" or "Tell me about _____" are, in general, unbiased as they allow clients to respond within their own frames of reference. Conversely, leading questions tend to encourage specific responses. For example, an interviewer might ask, "Based on our conversation, do you see why I am suggesting this hearing aid?" or "Based on these findings, when would you like to enroll for therapy?"

There are times when a leading question may be appropriate; for example, when we truly feel that someone should enroll for services, complete home activities suggested, or follow through with a referral being made. However, there are other times when a question with bias is inappropriate such as when trying to collect certain aspects of a case history or understand a patient's real feelings about a subject. Leading questions make honesty difficult when they lead interviewees to respond in ways that differ from their true feelings.

Reporters' Questions

Many interviewers and counselors also find it useful to distinguish between questions in the manner used by journalists. The well-known *wh* questions—*who, what, when, where, how,* and *why*—as well as *is* or *was, could,* and *should* all produce different types of responses. Ivey (1994) offers the following comments:

Who is the client? What is the client's personal background? Who else may be involved?

What is the client's problem? What is happening? What are the specific details of the situation?

When does the problem occur? When did it begin? What immediately preceded the occurrence of the problem?

Where does the problem occur? In what environments and situations?

How does the client react to the problem? How does the client feel about it?

Why does the problem occur?

> *Needless to say, the **who, what, when, where, how, why** series of questions also provides the interviewer with a ready system for helping the client elaborate or be more specific on an issue at any time during a session.... Often, but not always, key question stems result in predictable outcomes.*
>
> ***What** questions most often lead to facts. "What happened?" "What are you going to do?"*
>
> ***How** questions often lead to a discussion about processes or sequences or to feelings. "How could that be explained?" "How do you feel about that?"*
>
> ***Why** questions most often lead to discussion of reasons. "Why did you allow that to happen?" "Why do you think that is so?"*
>
> ***Could** questions are considered maximally open and contain some of the advantages of closed questions in that the client is free to say "No, I don't want to talk about that." Could questions reflect less control and command than others. "Could you tell me more about your situation?" "Could you give me a specific example?" "Could you tell me what you'd like to talk about today?"* (p. 56)

As described here, different questions do result in different types of information being discussed. Interviewers should be particularly careful when asking *why* questions because they put many respondents on the defensive. Why questions may also be perceived as prying, or they may engender feelings of guilt (Dillard & Reilly, 1988c). *Is* or *was* questions can also present problems by putting interviewees on the spot. A good alternative is to use *could* questions, which tend to be less judgmental and more tentative. Consider questions like "Was the car traveling too fast?" versus "Could the car have been traveling too fast?" The could question is more tentative, suggesting the possibility without requiring an absolute commitment of "yes" or "no." Could questions also provide interviewees with some degree of freedom and control in an interview. For example, if asked, "Could you tell me more about that?" the interviewee might feel free to say, "I really don't have anything more to add." For these reasons, could questions can be very useful in clinical interviewing and counseling (Shipley & Wood, 1996).

The question categories that have been discussed here—open or closed, primary or secondary, neutral or leading, and the *wh* or reporters' questions are not mutually exclusive. Any particular question asked can be open and neutral, open and leading, open and primary, closed and neutral, closed and leading, and so forth. Any combination is possible in the framing of questions. Interviewers just need to be aware that each question type has a different use and that the different combinations will evoke different responses. Figure 4.1 can be useful for interviewers to identify the types of questions they ask during interviews.

Question Feedback Sheet

_____ (Date)

_____   _____
(Name of Interviewer)   (Name of Person Completing Form)

Instructions: List below as completely as possible the questions asked by the interviewer. At a minimum, indicate the first key words of the question
(what, why, how, are, and so on). Indicate whether each question was
open (O) or closed (C).

_____   1. _____

_____   2. _____

_____   3. _____

_____   4. _____

_____   5. _____

_____   6. _____

_____   7. _____

_____   8. _____

_____   9. _____

_____   10. _____

1. Which questions seemed to provide the most useful client information?

2. Provide specific feedback on the attending skills of the interviewer.

3. Cite your impressions of the interview.

FIGURE 4.1   Sample Interviewer Checklist

Source: From Allen L. Ivey, _Intentional Interviewing and Counseling: Facilitating Client Development in a Multicultural Society_ (3rd edition), p. 66. Copyright © 1994 Brooks/Cole Publishing
Company, a division of International Thomson Publishing Inc., Pacific Grove, CA 93950. Reprinted by
permission of the publisher.

The Sequencing of Questions

Stewart and Cash (1994) describe four general sequences of questions in interviews. Two of these are seen in many speech and hearing interactions—the funnel sequence and the inverted funnel sequence. The *funnel sequence* begins with more general, open questions and proceeds to more closed types of questions. The entire interview can proceed in this fashion as the general area becomes more and more specific across the discussion. Or, more commonly, a funnel sequence is used for each new primary question before moving on to the next primary question. The *inverted-funnel sequence* moves in the opposite manner—from very specific, closed questions to more open questions. In general, a funnel sequence (from open to closed) is used most frequently in information-getting interviews. As Chapter 6 discusses, both sequences are used in information-giving interviews. A funnel approach is more useful in certain information-giving interviews; an inverted funnel approach works better in others.

Behaviors in an Interaction

Interviewing in particular is often thought of mainly as an exchange of specific information, in a question-and-response form. However, there is more to an effective interview than simply determining the right questions to ask or comments to share and then wording these verbalizations skillfully. There are, in fact, a number of verbal and nonverbal behaviors that can enhance or disrupt communication during interviewing and counseling sessions. These include verbal behaviors, vocal behaviors, nonverbal behaviors, and combinations of these. For purposes here, they are discussed under the headings of verbal behavior, nonverbal behavior, and other. Although these behavior types are considered individually here, clinicians usually employ them in combination with each other.

Verbal Behaviors

Encouragers. Encouragers are described in most texts dealing with effective interviewing and counseling (Donaghy, 1990; Ivey, 1994, Moursund, 1993; Okun, 1992; Stewart & Cash, 1994; and many others). These behaviors signal an interviewee to continue talking about the subject under discussion (Ivey, 1994; Johnson, 1988; Keane & Verman, 1985; Meier & Davis, 1993; Okun, 1992). There are many examples of verbal and vocal encouragers—saying "fine," "I see," "that's helpful," "good," "yes," and "keep going," or vocalizations such as "mmm" or "uh-huh."

Using these encouragers serves to increase patients' amounts of verbalization, decrease their times of silence, nurture positive client feelings toward clinicians, and help behaviors and attitudes that are encouraged generalize outside the interview or counseling situation. In operant terms, encouragers are social reinforcers. Some years ago, Richardson, Dohrenwend, and Klein (1965) provided an excellent discussion of the uses and effects of encouragements in interviewing. They commented that when encouragements are used purposefully and near the end of interviewee utterances, interviewees are more verbal and discuss a wider range of the topics of interest to interviewers. It is important to develop and use encouragers in interviewing and counseling because of their powerful effects in influencing client behavior. Effective and experienced counselors use encouragers significantly more often than ineffective or inexperienced counselors (Pederson & Ivey, 1993).

Orientations.   Orientations are verbalizations that provide direction or structure to interviews and counseling sessions. Examples of orientations include specific instructions or directions, explanatory statements, summaries, and paraphrases. Orientations can occur at any time during an interview.

Authorities on interviewing and counseling (Garrett, 1982; Lang, van der Molen, Trower, & Look, 1990; Martin & Hiebert, 1985; Stewart & Cash, 1994) advocate beginning an interaction with a clear statement of the purposes of the meeting—and concluding it with a summary of the major points discussed and a clear indication of future activities. However, direction and structure should also be provided before an interaction, as well as at the beginning, during, and at the end of an interview.

Preinterview or precounseling orientations provide clients with a sense of what to expect during the encounter. They let interviewees know the purposes of an interaction, at least generally what to expect, and approximately how long it might take (Shipley & Wood, 1996). Without such orientations, some clients may experience unnecessary uncertainty, concern, and anxiety about a forthcoming encounter. Clients who are given fairly complete information about what to expect tend to engage in more discussion of personal matters than clients who do not receive such information (Doster, 1972). It has also been found that patients tend to be less cooperative and to terminate services earlier when their expectations for an interview differ from what actually occurs (Clemes & D'Andrea, 1965). These factors—potentially discussing less personal information, less cooperation, and terminating earlier—are important reasons to consider providing appropriate presession orientations to clients and/or their caregivers.

Once a session actually begins, clinicians use orientations to direct or redirect areas of discussion. The characteristics of any interview depend, in large part, on the interviewer's structuring. The interviewer's instructions and directions define the areas to be explored. *Instructions* help interviewees understand what is expected of them, and how to proceed. *Directions* tell the client what to do or talk about next, or what actions are necessary (Ivey, 1994). Directions or instructions do not have to be complicated or long; for example, interviewers could use the following:

"I'd like you to tell me about how the stuttering developed."

"Talk about what the doctor said. Then we'll address what you are doing at home."

"I want you to call the teacher this week and discuss _____ ."

Some care should be given to how directive a direction really is, particularly with some multicultural clients. Among some cultures (e.g., Filipino or Japanese), very direct, command-like statements can be offensive. A more subtly worded request is preferable with such clients. *Explanations* describe how and why certain information or activities are necessary, thus helping clients understand requests or suggestions. Explaining why some types of information are needed is particularly helpful with more sensitive or personal subjects. *Summaries* and *paraphrases* clarify topics of discussion and signal that interviewees are being heard and understood. They act to stimulate interviewees' verbalizations within areas of interest to interviewers. Summaries and paraphrases also help ensure that clinicians understand information correctly; clients can correct any information that may have been misunderstood or misinterpreted. A summary or a paraphrase also acts as a transition point when clinicians want to move on to other discussion topics. Clinicians summarize or paraphrase what has just been discussed, then introduce the new topic for discussion.

Orientations structure and focus conversations. They introduce what should be discussed, encourage keeping on the tasks at hand, and lessen the chances of digressing into irrelevant topics. When a digression does occur, orientations are useful to get the discussion back "on track."

High- and low-specificity stimuli. Open and closed questions were described earlier in this chapter. Closed questions are examples of high specificity stimuli—the question itself requires a rather specific type of response, or a high degree of specificity. Open questions are just the opposite, allowing interviewers to field these questions in a number of ways. Thus, there is a low level of specificity required. Like questions, directives are also high or low in the level of specificity required. Consider the following examples:

"Tell me about some of your concerns." (low specificity)

"Describe your conversation with _____ ." (high specificity)

Open, low-specificity stimuli result in longer responses that cover a wider range of topics. Closed stimuli result in shorter, more focused responses (Brammer, 1993; Dainow & Bailey, 1988; Woolf, 1971). Open and closed stimuli, whether questions or directives, are used at different times during a discussion. For example, when specific information is needed about the chronology of a problem, clinicians may use a closed stimulus ("Tell me about the ear infections"). But if the events of that particular time period then need to be discussed, clinicians can use a more open stimulus ("Three months ago? What was going on three months ago?").

Interpretations.   Interpretations are verbalizations that describe *why* behaviors, events, or feelings have occurred. They are aimed at providing new perspectives for a client's consideration (Brammer, 1993). In a psychological sense, interpretations are used to help provide meaning for dreams, thoughts, or behaviors (Lang et al., 1990). However, interpretations are sometimes used to get at other kinds of realities—physical, social, spiritual—expressed by feelings, symptoms, and behaviors. The following are basic principles for using interpretations.

1. Look for the interviewee's basic message.
2. Provide the interviewee with a paraphrase of what you think a message means.
3. Convey your understanding of what the message means in terms of your theory or your general explanation of motives, defenses, and needs.
4. Keep your language simple and similar to that used by the interviewee. Avoid wild speculation and statements in esoteric wording.
5. Use statements that indicate you are offering tentative ideas about what the client's words or behaviors mean. "Is this a fair statement?" "The way I see it is _____." "I wonder if _____."
6. Solicit interviewees' reactions to your interpretations.
7. Teach interviewees to do their own interpreting. You cannot give insight to others; they must make their own discoveries. (Adapted from Brammer, 1993, p. 95.)

Some cautions are in order regarding the use of interpretations. First, bear in mind that interpretation is based on an individual clinician's expertise, experience, insight, and personal frame of reference. It is possible that another clinician would formulate an alternative interpretation. The accuracy of a particular interpretation can be culturally related. For example, it is relatively common in U.S. culture to view extended silence as a potential sign of anger, resentment, disagreement, confusion, or lack of understanding. However, extended periods of silence during interactions are within normal communicative expectations in some Middle Eastern cultures (Irujo, 1988). Silence, which a clinician might interpret as a possible indication of noncooperation, resentment, hostility, or even the withholding of information, may simply be a normal communicative style with some individuals from these cultures. Second, remember that psychologically based interpretations are beyond the boundaries of the training and experience of most speech-language pathologists or audiologists. Finally, realize that interpretations have powerful effects that tend to inhibit clients' immediate verbalizations and that the memory of having been interpreted may remain a factor in future interviews (Brammer, 1993; Kanfer, Phillips, Matarazzo, & Saslow, 1960).

The act of interpreting why something has occurred can significantly, and sometimes negatively, affect an interaction. This may occur irrespective of whether the interpretation was actually correct or incorrect. The point is, be careful with the use of interpretations. Clinicians need to be aware of these verbalizations and not use them inadvertently.

Evaluations. Evaluations are positive or negative judgments and comments about someone's actions, behavior, feelings, statements, or questions. They are needed in many instances; for example, when providing feedback about the mastery of some target behavior or when evaluating someone's assistance with generalization efforts. However, even when evaluations are necessary and offered for the right reasons, they can still inhibit or shorten interviewees' and counselees' responses immediately following the evaluation (Johns, 1975). A conventional expectation is that positive evaluations should increase a client's verbalization. In actuality, however, an evaluative comment—whether positive or negative—typically inhibits interviewees' subsequent verbalization. This phenomenon is similar in some ways to receiving a compliment. Many individuals, while pleased, say little other than "Thank you" or "Thank you—I'm glad you like it" immediately following such a positive evaluation.

There are instances in which patients or families may view certain evaluative statements as demonstrating a lack of interviewer sincerity and understanding, or as evidence that an interviewer is acting in a superior or judgmental manner (Powell, 1968). The emergence of such feelings is particularly possible with some clients from linguistically and culturally diverse backgrounds that differ from the clinician's. Clinicians would be remiss if they did not provide appropriate evaluative comments as needed in their clinical work. However, they also need to realize the possible effects some evaluations may have so they can use them constructively and not be surprised by their effects.

Neutral or social verbalizations. Verbalizations that do not relate directly to an interview and its purposes are referred to as neutral or social. Perhaps the most common example of a neutral or social comment is what Molyneaux and Lane (1982) have called "nonpertinent small talk." Such small talk might include comments about the weather, about difficulties finding parking, or about what the participants did for recreation over the weekend. Several observational and self-analysis systems used to study clinical treatment in communicative disorders have included sections that look at clinicians' neutral or social verbalizations (e.g., Boone & Prescott, 1972; Molyneaux & Lane, 1982; Prescott & Tesauro, 1974). It is important to identify the presence of these behaviors because, when used excessively, they do reduce overall effectiveness in clinical sessions.

Neutral and social comments do not typically relate directly to the tasks at hand, so too many of them take up important time. Rache, Bernstein, and Veenhuis (1974) studied the interviewing skills of medical students and found that "social conversation skills...must be replaced by responsible communication if the [physician-patient] relationship is to be productive" (p. 591). They also commented that unless medical students received specific training in interviewing, they tended to use too many social comments, to the relative exclusion of more purposeful or insightful interaction. The same holds true for students learning to work with communicative disorders.

Still, neutral or social comments are not always inappropriate. For example, a brief period of social conversation is often helpful when two parties are beginning to establish a relationship. Similarly, two parties who have interacted before may have a relationship that calls for more than "getting right down to business." These brief periods of exchanging socials pleasantries (called *platicando* in the Hispanic culture) are important prerequisites to further interaction. However, neutral and social interactions do need to be controlled. The interviewer should strive to use them only as vehicles for increasing patient comfort and interview communication. There is usually little, if any, need for such conversations once a meeting is underway; those that occur during an interaction generally signal that the participants are off task.

Nonverbal Behaviors

A number of nonverbal behaviors have a demonstrated effect on interview communication (Burgoon, 1994; Edinger & Patterson, 1983; Mehrabian, 1972; Siegman & Feldstein, 1987). Whether they realize it or not, interviewers and counselors influence their interactions by using nonverbal behaviors such as facial expressions, head nodding, specific leans and postures of the body, eye contact, and touching the other party.

Facial expression.   Facial expressions convey anger, disgust, fear, sadness, or happiness (Hackney & Cormier, 1994). They also can convey agreement, disagreement, surprise, or even confusion or bewilderment. There are a number of potentially important feelings and messages conveyed by facial expression. Scheuerle (1992) considers facial expression to be as important as eye contact in maintaining interpersonal communication. There are many possible messages communicated by facial expressions, many of which can reveal possible insights into clients' reactions to information discussed and their inner feelings about subjects discussed. Careful observation of the facial area can be important.

Positive and negative head nodding. Head nodding is a communicative event—it communicates a message (Dittman, 1987; Thompson, 1973). Vertical, up-and-down head nods indicate pleasure, approval, or agreement in the Western culture. Horizontal, or side-to-side, nods suggest displeasure, disapproval, or disagreement. But this is not the case across all cultures. Russians, for example, nod in just the opposite fashion—up-and-down indicates "no" and side-to-side suggests "yes" (Ivey, 1994).

Head nods, whether positive or negative, tend to occur in combination with other behaviors, such as statements of approval or disapproval and accompanying facial expressions. There is a considerable amount of evidence to suggest that head nodding, particularly in combination with other behaviors, influences interviewees' verbal behavior during interviewing and counseling (Burgoon, 1994; Fretz, 1966; Mehrabian, 1972; Rosenfeld, 1967). Unless they are overused, positive head nods communicate that an interviewer is attending, convey a liking attitude toward the other party, and signal interviewees to keep talking. Positive nods are also associated with truthfulness, although this can be deceptive. Conversely, negative nodding acts to discourage or inhibit communication. They indicate that information is not being understood, that there is disagreement with something said, or that the topic of discussion should not be pursued further. Negative nodding also can be interpreted as being judgmental.

Clinicians should use head nodding purposefully to communicate those messages they wish to convey—agreement, keep on talking, disagreement, and so forth. Many clinicians, particularly those who are beginning or are less effective, are not aware of their use of head nods. These are powerful behaviors that need to be used consciously and purposefully.

Body posturing and leaning. Body leaning and the general posturing of people in interview situations is one indicator of what is happening during an exchange (Shipley & Wood, 1996). A postural shift can be important not so much as personality indicators but as communicative events (Scheflen, 1964). The postural change discussed most frequently in interviewing and counseling literature is leaning the body forward or backward. Forward leans usually indicate interest, affirmative response, and respect and liking. Therefore, they are presumed to facilitate communication. Backward leans, on the other hand, are considered signs of disinterest, negative response, and unfavorable feelings, and they tend to inhibit interviewee verbalizations and communication (Mehrabian, 1972). Like head nods, body leans tend not to occur by themselves but in combination with positive or negative head nods and comments.

Many clinicians purposefully lean forward to indicate interest or when making a point they feel is important. Similarly, many interviewers and counselors carefully observe patients' body leans as an indication of their interest or agreement within areas of discussion, and as a way to try to judge how well information is being received. Culture, however, plays a role in interpreting what body postures actually indicate. For example, in some Appalachian communities, a relaxed, backward, "belly first" posture is associated with genuine interest, whereas a forward-leaning posture suggests that the other party may be somewhat unnerved (Keefe, 1988).

Eye contact.   It is generally agreed that "good eye contact" facilitates communication in interviewing and counseling situations (Cormier & Hackney, 1987; Ivey, 1994). However, the frequency and even the duration of eye contact reflect other factors besides just the quality of a relationship and any communication that is occurring. Eye contact is related to such factors as the genders of the participants; either party's attitude toward the other party; the participants' attraction to each other; the participants' personalities; the decor of the setting; and, of course, the nature of any verbal and nonverbal communication that is happening (Donaghy, 1990; Kleinke, Staneski, & Berger, 1975; Libby & Yaklevich, 1973; Rosenfeld & Civikly, 1976; Shipley & Wood, 1996).

The use of eye contact is very much culturally related. Direct eye contact during communication is characteristic of white middle-class culture in the United States. African Americans tend to use more eye contact when talking and less when listening. Some African American children will make little eye contact with adults because it is considered disrespectful (Tiegerman-Farber, 1995). Among some Hispanic and Asian groups, eye contact by the young is also considered disrespectful and is therefore discouraged (Ivey, 1994; Roseberry-McKibbin, 1995; Sue, 1988). Many Muslim males do not establish eye contact with females or, to show respect, avert their gaze (Nellum-Davis, 1993). There are many other examples that could be noted.

Eye contact is important to consider, but it interacts with many other variables. Thus, guard against overinferring information solely by the presence or absence of eye contact. The interviewer should strive to maintain good eye contact, but not to a degree that an interviewee feels stared at, feels under constant inspection, or feels violated.

Touch.   Touching an interviewee or their caregiver can have positive effects on a relationship and the communication that occurs within it, or it can have damaging effects on a relationship and any subsequent communication. This depends on when and where a touch is given, and how the other party perceives it (Shipley & Wood, 1996). Touch in the form of hand shaking is a customary way of welcoming people, of expressing pleasure at meeting and getting to know them. At the close of a meeting, a handshake can indicate enjoyment of or satisfaction with the encounter. Shaking hands also can indicate the desire to continue a relationship even though discussions have included disagreement. However, some handshakes can be interpreted in different ways. A warm and somewhat firm handshake with appropriate distance between the parties can appear appropriately "businesslike," but a "more intimate" handshake with too little distance or by clasping both hands can be perceived as being too personal for some individuals. There are also cultural nuances to a handshake. Males from certain cultures (e.g., some Middle Eastern cultures) may interpret a handshake from a female as being forward, inappropriate, or even in a sexual manner. Of course, how a handshake is done can be interpreted differently across a number of cultures.

There are other cultural factors to consider when touching someone else. Touching the head, particularly with children, is discomforting for many individuals from Asian, Carolinian, Chamorro, and a number of other cultures (Hammer, 1994; Buell, 1985; Roseberry-McKibbin, 1995). Within the context of these considerations, however, touching in nonintimate, friendly ways can express warmth or understanding during interviewing and counseling sessions irrespective of the gender of the participants (Kleinke, 1986). For example, a caring touch on the shoulder or on the back of the hand can help express empathy and concern to someone in distress. Such touching can help to increase client willingness to interact and communicate with the clinician. However, a touch that is interpreted as being more intimate or sexual in nature can seriously impair or even destroy a good working relationship. One question clinicians need to ask themselves is whether a touch is used for the client or for themselves. If there is any doubt about the purpose of a touch, the touch should be avoided (Moursund, 1985). It is important to remember that any touching needs to be done in a fashion that cannot be perceived as being sexual or too personal in nature.

Other Behaviors

Silences. Periods of silence during a conversation are very acceptable within some cultures (e.g., the Arabic culture), but less acceptable in others. In the general U.S. culture, silence during conversation can be disconcerting, particularly when two parties are just getting acquainted. Silence is feared by many interviewers—they may feel awkward, lost, or out of control. Periods of silence can express several distinct realities. Silence can result from poor interviewing skills, from poorly framed questions, or indecision. Silence can occur when individuals feel "stumped" or surprised by something said, are unsure of what direction to take next, or are uncomfortable that nothing is happening at the moment. Unfortunately, many people's inclination is to say something to break a silence; often, this is the worst thing to do.

Hackney and Cormier (1994) offer the following comments about counselors and silence:

> *For most beginning counselors, silence can be frightening. It seems to bring the total focus of attention on them, revealing their most glaring weaknesses as counselors—at least this is how many beginning counselors describe their experiences with silence. Typically a question is asked. Often it is a bad question—one that can be answered by a minimal response from the client. The answer to the question is relatively unimportant, since the question was not well thought out by the counselor. The counselor may not even be listening to the answer.* (p. 50)

Many times, such periods of silence are best not interrupted prematurely. Exercise discipline and decide how to respond rather than responding too quickly with something that is not particularly productive or may actually compound the problem.

There is another type of *silence*—which is a powerful, purposefully used clinical technique that is meant to affect communication in interviewing and counseling sessions. These silences are periods of time when interviewers purposely withhold their verbalizations or vocalizations as a signal for interviewees to respond, to begin speaking, or to resume speaking (Moursund, 1993; Richardson et al., 1965; Shipley & Wood, 1996). Silences that are relatively short (generally about 5 seconds or less) and that are terminated by an interviewee will act to increase the length of the interviewee's verbalizations. They signal the person to begin or to continue talking about a subject area. The use of short, purposeful silences helps the interviewee for the following reasons:

- Many respondents may need time to formulate their thoughts or determine their response. If a clinician does not remain silent during that time, the respondent's thoughts and subsequent verbalizations are inhibited.
- Even when interviewees think they have completed the expression of some thought, an interviewer's use of a purposeful silence indicates that they should continue along that line of thought or expand further.
- Finding the silence uncomfortable, respondents may continue by either elaborating on the previous subject or introducing a new topic. Silence thus acts to make the interviewee more responsible for providing additional information or new directions in interview situations.

There are some limitations to silence. Silences that last much longer than about 5 seconds (e.g., 10-15 seconds) are likely to be terminated by the interviewer, and result in shorter verbalizations from interviewees. The excessive use of silences, such as to the point that interviewees begin to feel that is all an interviewer is doing, is also counterproductive. Clients can resent this use of silence. However, when used correctly, purposeful silence is a powerful and useful clinical tool.

Interruptions and "guggles." In the white U.S. culture, it is considered rude to interrupt someone who is speaking. Interruptions can have powerful effects such as creating agitation, cutting off the other person, and even inhibiting further attempts to communicate. One study found that the more interviewees were subjected to interruptions, the less interactive they became (Phillips, Matarazzo, Matarazzo, Saslow, & Kanfer, 1961). Other cultures have similar values; for example, among some Asians, interruptions in a conversation may be considered very impolite and inappropriate. Among some African Americans, however, certain conversations may become competitive, with the most assertive speaker doing most of the talking. If a participant feels a need to add information, an interruption or change of topic may occur (Roseberry-McKibbin, 1995).

In general, interviewers and counselors need to control their use of interruptions. However, this does not mean that interruptions should always be avoided. Interruptions can be used purposefully with certain highly verbal patients, or in cases where a redirection of the conversation is needed. Emerick (1969) provides an excellent example of a case when an interruption, indeed multiple interruptions, would be appropriate:

> *Mrs. Griewe was an attractive but rather harried mother of six children, all under nine years of age. Her four-year-old daughter, Mary, was beginning to stutter, and Mrs. Griewe came to the clinic for assistance. The longer she talked, the more she talked about herself, rather than the child. Finally, she broke down and said that her problem was her religion, a faith which forbade birth control, but as she pointed out ruefully, did not assist with the child-rearing duties. She revealed that she had a college degree but it was of no use since she operated on the level of diapers and runny noses year after year. She blurted out a lot of other things about the clergy and the trap she felt she was in. I tried desperately to shut off the flow but could not. I never saw Mary again.* (p. 26)

The problem in this case is that the interviewee revealed too much too quickly—well before a firm relationship had been established. Had the patient-clinician relationship been more fully established, the two parties might have stayed in contact for an eventual referral for the counseling help needed. Also, the child might have obtained the help she needed for the fluency problem. This example helps illustrate how an interruption, or in this particular case several interruptions, could be appropriate and necessary. Sometimes, in cases like this example, literally interrupting the other party or asking a series of closed questions in a rapid fashion can be ways of disrupting a patient's or caregiver's flow of discussion.

The term *guggles* has been used to describe interruptive devices, which are less powerful and less offensive than overt interruptions, but still act to interrupt or redirect conversation (Richardson et al., 1965). Guggles can be verbal, vocal, or nonverbal. They serve to signal an interviewee that "it's my turn to talk" or that some redirection is desired. Clinicians might clear the throat or interject a short "ah" during a client's verbalization. Such vocal behaviors interrupt or signal interviewees in a covert manner. Clinicians can also use physical movements like glancing toward a window, checking the time, taking a deep breath, or shuffling papers as cues for changing or terminating a conversation (Knapp, 1972). Of course, some subtlety is needed when using guggles or they can appear rude.

Encouragers were discussed earlier in this chapter as examples of verbal behaviors that facilitate and encourage communication. The question arises, what if encouragers are used too frequently or are introduced too early during an interviewee's utterance? In such cases, what a clinician intends as an encourager actually inhibits or discourages interviewees' verbalizations and their overall levels of communication. Consider how the timing of an interviewer's "I see" affects an interviewee's utterance in the following examples:

> *CLIENT:* When he was about three years old, he started to read and really enjoyed the attention he got from us each night.
> *CLINICIAN:* I see.

> *CLIENT:* When he was about three years old . . .
> *CLINICIAN:* I see.

The timing in the first example would encourage the interviewee to continue discussing this or a related topic. However, the premature timing in the second instance interrupts what is being expressed; it would inhibit the interviewee from completing the utterance and probably discourage further discussion of the topic. Thus, the same phrase (a simple "I see") can be an encouragement or a guggle depending on how and when it is used.

Guggles do not reduce overall interviewee participation if used sparingly and with some subtlety; however, the premature or frequent use of guggles or interruptions will be perceived as rudeness, which results in less interviewee participation (Richardson et al., 1965; Shipley & Wood, 1996). Interruptions and guggles should be used consciously and purposefully. Many people are not fully aware of their use of interruptions and guggles and are therefore affecting other people's communication without even realizing it. It is important for interviewers to be aware of their own verbal, vocal, and nonverbal actions—and to control them!

Several Fundamental Techniques

Summaries, reflections, clarifications, repetitions, pauses, confrontations, and appropriate types of self-disclosure are techniques that utilize some of the verbal and nonverbal behaviors described in this chapter. These techniques can facilitate communication during interviewing and counseling sessions in a number of ways.

Summaries

Clinicians use summaries and reflections to feed back the essential elements of a client's comments. Summaries facilitate communication by signaling that information expressed by the client has been heard and understood; they mirror back the messages, attitudes, and feelings the client has expressed (Dillard & Reilly, 1988c; Ivey, 1994). A summary also helps highlight the major points made by an interviewer. A good summary uses the clinician's own words, rather than the interviewee's words, and captures the most important topics discussed—essentially hitting the "high spots."

Summaries during an interaction keep a discussion moving by encouraging interviewees to explore topics and attitudes in greater detail (Mowrer, 1988). They are also used so both interviewers and patients can "double-check" that the clinician is understanding what the other party is really saying.

Interviewers use summaries at the end of an interview to wrap up or terminate discussion. A good closing summary highlights the major points discussed and helps the interviewee feel that the parties have accomplished a purpose. This also helps interviewees to leave feeling that they have been understood—or at least listened to attentively (Purkey & Schmidt, 1987).

Reflections

Reflections are typically shorter than summaries and stick closely to the very words interviewees have used to express their thoughts or feelings. When employing reflections, interviewers should avoid projecting their own opinions and feelings into the comments (Brammer, 1993). There are three basic types of reflections: (1) reflection of the content of the client's message, (2) reflection of both the content of the message and the feelings the client has expressed about the content, (3) short reflection (or "accentuation")—restatement of key words or phrases as questions ("Pain?" "Stuttering?").

Reflections are effective in helping to check whether the clinician has correctly understood and interpreted any information presented. They also serve to promote further discussion within the area. Often greater understanding occurs for both parties as interviewees or counselees respond to a reflection.

Clarifications

Interviewers and counselors use clarifications to more fully understand a client and the client's difficulties (Schuyler & Rushmer, 1987). When something is confusing or ambiguous, interviewers use a clarification to specify the area of confusion. The interviewer might say, for example, "Tell me more about your father's speech problem" or "What do you mean when you say your child's speech sounds immature?" When clinicians need to clarify a larger segment of information, a summary may be in order. "Let me review what I think you are saying _____."

Like summaries, clarifications help clinicians understand the content of a client's topic and also the client's feelings about the subject. Clarifications can be used to find out more about specific behavior or to exchange perceptions regarding what has been said. A tentatively expressed clarification gives clients an opportunity to agree or disagree and to add additional information. Beginning a clarification, the clinician might ask, "Did I understand you correctly when you said that _____?" Such a question can facilitate further clarification if there has been confusion or miscommunication.

Repetitions

Clinicians are frequently in the situation of trying to maintain interviewees' attention (Nirenberg, 1968). An interviewee's attention can vacillate between what an interviewer is saying and what the individual is thinking about at that moment. For example, an interviewee who is thinking about the costs of therapy may miss a clinician's "beautifully worded" description of the communicative problem. The dangers of "drifting" are especially great when interviewees are tired or tense, when there are distractions, or when they must make difficult decisions requiring careful consideration.

Clinicians cannot assume that an interviewee's complete attention can be maintained at all times—virtually everyone's attention drifts periodically. However, the purposeful use of repetitions helps provide sufficient redundance to enable interviewees to grasp the basic message even if they have missed some particular comments. The words that clients do hear and process may carry enough meaning to effectively communicate the clinician's thoughts. For this reason, deliberate repetitions are extremely useful in interviewing and counseling conversations.

Although repetition in writing is often viewed with disapproval, judicious repetition is essential for effective oral communication in interviewing and counseling sessions. Repetitions help the speaker to avoid losing the listener—the more often information is heard, the more it tends to be understood and retained. The speaker who uses repetition in this way can achieve clarity and emphasis while helping listeners catch more of the message. When using repetitions, clinicians hold an interviewee's interest and avoid the appearance of repeating themselves by varying their wordings each time and, when appropriate, giving bits of additional information with each subsequent repetition (Mowrer, 1988). Planned repetitions are very useful when working with some individuals for whom there are language barriers, and for whom the material being covered is unfamiliar. They are also helpful when working with an interpreter present.

Pauses

A *pause* is a very brief moment of silence. Pauses during a session provide people with opportunities to ponder and reflect (Moursund, 1993). They do the same for clinicians; brief pauses can be helpful to either party. Because pausing does suggest that one is thinking, interviewers who fail to employ pauses may be inadvertently suggesting to some interviewees that their statements are not being taken seriously. Clinicians, therefore, are well advised to pause occasionally, even if such pausing is not necessary for the formulation of questions or responses.

Pausing is more natural in some cultures than in others. In the white U.S. culture, a pause is a period of silence and therefore it can be somewhat disconcerting to many individuals. Among many native American groups, etiquette requires a lapse of time between a question and an answer. Some native Americans feel that if a question is answered too quickly, it may not have been worth thinking about in the first place (Gilliland, 1992).

Confrontations

The word "confrontation" tends to conjure up images of something mean-spirited or hostile, but this is not what is meant by confrontation in interviewing and counseling. Confrontations are very powerful techniques that do, however, enable clients to face and deal with realities, situations, and behaviors that they are inclined to avoid or deny (Brammer, 1993; Cormier & Hackney, 1987; Pederson & Ivey, 1993). Brammer (1993) describes the basic aspects of confrontation:

> *The idea of confronting is to recognize honestly and directly and to point out to helpees what is going on or what you infer is going on. The effects are challenge, exposure, or threat. Resulting emotional effects are sometimes anxiety when challenged with feedback from the helper, and sometimes pleasure with his or her honest opinions and expressions of caring. In other words, confronting skills, involve risk—resulting either in unwanted resistance from helpees or in desired openness of communication.* (p. 83)

Clinicians should use confrontation purposefully in a careful manner that expresses empathy for patients and concern for their best interests. An especially accepting tone of voice may be needed (Lang et al., 1990). Mowrer (1988) provides this rather direct example of confrontation with a high school student:

Bill has discussed advantages and disadvantages of enrolling in a high school speech class to work on his falsetto voice. He is making no special progress toward a decision so you might say, "Well, Bill, it's up to you, do you want to enroll or not?" or "You've been beating around the bush, Bill, why can't you make up your mind? Is it that you feel like a grade-school kid coming to speech class?" (p. 399)

A "you said _____ but _____" construction is often used with a confrontation; for example:

"You said you really needed the help, but you have missed your last two appointments."

"You said you would get the medical clearance, but you haven't gotten it yet."

"You said that you cannot make a good /r/, but listen to the tape."

The discussion of discrepancies and mixed messages in Chapter 9 includes several other confrontation formats.

Confrontation is an important tool in the professional's repertoire. However, if not used skillfully and appropriately, it can be a blunt instrument that is harmful to patients and to the patient-professional relationships (Kennedy, 1977). Confrontational techniques should never be used to punish or as expressions of hostility or anger. Confrontation is properly a facilitative technique used to engender greater understanding or necessary action. If clinicians have doubts about their motives or about the appropriateness of the technique in a given situation, if clinicians cannot reasonably estimate a client's response, and/or if clinicians are working with an emotionally unstable person, using a confrontation may be unwise. Clinicians should also bear in mind that overusing this technique can make some clients feel like they are being criticized or nagged.

Self-Disclosure

Interviewers and counselors practice self-disclosure when they share some of their personal experiences or feelings with their clients. The judicious use of self-disclosure conveys empathy and support to clients and caregivers (McDonald & Haney, 1988), or it lets them see that the clinician is "really a person" rather than just someone in a role (Cormier & Hackney, 1987; Hackney & Cormier, 1994). Disclosing something about ourselves can be useful in the overall development of a relationship. Some clients, particularly certain individuals from diverse backgrounds, feel better about a relationship if they know something about the clinician. In attempting to get to know the clinician better, individuals from some groups (e.g., the Filipino culture) may even ask what are perceived as being rather personal questions—(Are you married? Do you have children? Why not?). Such questions are not being rudely asked; rather, they are a means of getting to know the clinician better. Appropriate levels of self-disclosure here can be helpful in facilitating rapport between the parties.

It is important to understand that self-disclosure is a clinical tool that can be used to help clients become more comfortable, to understand particular concepts, to experience empathy that the clinician is feeling, and to understand that clinicians are people. Self-disclosure is not unguided, purposeless, or self-serving talk about the clinician and events in his or her life. Whether some specific self-disclosure is appropriate (i.e., whether it is done on behalf of the client rather than the clinician) usually depends on the answer to the following question: "Whose needs am I meeting—the client's or mine?" (Hackney & Cormier, 1979). Self-disclosure to meet the client's needs is an appropriate facilitating technique; self-disclosure to meet the clinician's needs is inappropriate self-indulgence.

Concluding Comments

An effective interviewer-counselor has a number of tools that affect the communication that occurs with others. These include several different kinds of questions and many specific behaviors and techniques that influence communication during interviewing and counseling situations. Verbal, vocal, and nonverbal behaviors are always involved in the communication process—whether we are conscious of them or not. They can either facilitate or impede the process. As interviewers become more conscious of and gain more control over these behaviors, they become invaluable tools for structuring, controlling, and providing direction to these interactions. The keys are a solid understanding of the various skills; good interactive skills; and, to borrow Haynes, Pindzola, and Emerick's (1992) words, "practice, practice, practice..."

C h a p t e r 5

Obtaining Information

Information-getting interviews are an integral part of the diagnostic and treatment process (Clark, 1994b, Haynes, Pindzola, & Emerick, 1992; Peterson & Marquardt, 1994; Shipley & McAfee, 1992). These interviews allow clinicians to gather appropriate information about clients, determine their present and past levels of functioning, identify various factors surrounding the case, and determine their potential for improvement. Thus, the functions of information-getting interviews include the following:

- Helping in the determination of whether a problem exists.
- Obtaining information that will aid in understanding the causes of a problem.
- Assessing factors related to the existence of a problem.
- Predicting future communicative abilities, with or without intervention.
- Developing appropriate treatment recommendations, goals, and procedures.

Successful informational interviews do not occur by accident or luck (Stewart, 1972). Rather, success occurs in the presence of effective interactional abilities, knowledge of interviewing techniques, skill in asking questions and obtaining information, careful listening, and a knowledge about communicative development and disorders. The absence of any of these qualities or skills can render any interview ineffective—or at least less effective than would otherwise be possible.

Clinicians typically use questions and probes to gather both objective and subjective types of information during information-getting interviews. Because these interviews are performed to gather information and a greater understanding of patients, they are not intended to alter or influence interviewees' behavior or attitudes. In fact, clinicians generally avoid trying to change an interviewee's feelings within these interview types. However, there are occasions during some information-getting interviews when the release and ventilation of patients' feelings and fears can positively change their behavior and attitudes (Darley, 1978; Haynes et al., 1992).

Orienting interviewees toward what to expect during an interview is a helpful prerequisite for these interviews. Then, once an interview begins, there are three stages or phases to this interaction: (1) an opening, (2) the body of the interview, and (3) the closing.

These are three distinct phases, which cover different types of information and differ in length. The most substantial information pertaining to the case is determined in the body of the interview. The discussions that follow address orienting an interviewee, then focus on the structure and content of the three phases of interviews to obtain information.

Presession Orientations

Providing Orientation Information

Clinicians set the stage for optimal success by providing presession orientations for interviewees. There are several ways to do this. In settings with support staff available, these individuals can inform patients about the services to be received. When clients contact an agency or facility to make an appointment, a knowledgeable administrator or assistant provides general information concerning the basic procedures involved, the professional who will be seen, any fees charged, the length of sessions, and so forth. Of course, support staff members will need to be trained to convey appropriate types of information to clients, their families, and other caregivers.

Another way to orient people is through direct client–clinician contact, typically by telephone. Clinicians can provide basic information concerning the agency or setting and the types of activities that will be involved. This also provides a good opportunity to answer various procedural or general questions clients may have. Such contacts are beneficial because clients and others in their environment are given an opportunity to speak briefly with the clinician prior to a first visit.

Presession orientations can also involve sending written information—a letter or pamphlet describing the setting, the services it provides, or general information about speech and hearing development or disorders. A note or card confirming the time and date of the appointment is also useful.

A case history form is frequently provided to patients or caregivers for completion prior to a first visit. The history form itself can help orient clients toward what may be discussed as medical, educational, social, or communicative histories are considered in completing the form. The form also helps clinicians obtain preliminary information about the client and, when returned in advance, it helps clinicians prepare for a session. A release-of-information form is sometimes sent to authorize requests for information from other professionals who have seen a client (Martin, 1994).

In addition to the specific information provided about the clinical setting, various pamphlets or brochures dealing with preparing for a first visit, specific communicative disorders (e.g., hearing loss, voice problems, cleft palate, stuttering), and communicative disorders in general are available. Such resources are available through professional organizations like the American Speech-Language-Hearing Association (ASHA), some state speech and hearing associations, many state licensing boards, and some commercial publishers in the field. Some of these items, particularly from ASHA, are available in different languages.

The use of such orienting procedures helps minimize clients' uncertainty or anxiety before an appointment, provides information about what will occur during the first visit, and helps engender overall levels of cooperation and rapport in many instances. However, there are some factors to consider before implementing these as "standard operating procedure." It does little good, and indeed may have some negative effects, when written materials that are provided cannot be read because of illiteracy, or the materials are written in an unfamiliar language. In some settings and locations, materials in different languages will be needed. Also, be aware that materials sent home with a child, such as from school, may lead caregivers from some backgrounds to an immediate assumption that the child has misbehaved or done something wrong. A clear explanation of what is being sent should precede the sending of such information.

Using an Appropriate Title or Salutation

A tentative relationship between clinicians and clients begins to develop before their first face-to-face meeting. Clients' perceptions of the setting as well as the practitioner's reputation and abilities influence their initial attitudes and behavior toward clinicians (Hartbauer, 1978; Moursund, 1993; Shipley & Wood, 1996).

The title a professional uses also can influence interviewees. Years ago, Gelso and Karl (1974) found that students judged professional counselors' skill levels differently on the basis of the titles they used. These investigators compared students' reactions to various titles—high school counselor, advisor, college counselor, counseling psychologist, clinical psychologist, and psychiatrist. Not surprisingly, they found that different titles created different initial perceptions. Those who were labeled counseling psychologists or clinical psychologists were perceived as being more knowledgeable than those using other titles. This is a factor in our field, particularly in speech-language pathology. Clinicians are sometimes referred to as speech pathologists, speech-language pathologists, speech clinicians, speech and hearing specialists, speech teachers, and so forth. It is helpful for clients to know how to refer to the clinician; clinicians should choose a professional title that is accurate, complies with current acceptable usage, and helps engender appropriate levels of respect.

Clinicians' use of their first name—or their last name preceded by Dr., Ms., Miss, Mrs., or Mr.—should also be considered carefully. There has been a trend in the general culture in the last three or four decades toward using first names more frequently than occurred earlier this century. However, many older individuals find this disconcerting when initially establishing a relationship, particularly with a clinician who is younger. Likewise, many individuals from linguistically and culturally diverse populations find the use of either party's first names, especially early in a relationship, inappropriate or disconcerting.

Occasionally, first-time clients with communicative disorders will inquire about the background of a clinician whom they are scheduled to see. Either support personnel or the clinician can provide a brief description of the professional credentials, depending on who is asked; for example:

> "You will be seeing Mr. Jones. He is a speech-language pathologist who has worked here with children for more than seven years. He has worked with many children who have stuttered."

> "Dr. Smith is our audiologist. She has her doctoral degree and more than ten years of experience with hearing and hearing problems. She works with many people who might benefit from hearing aids."

> "I am Ms. Vang. I am the speech pathologist who will be seeing Vanessa. I finished my degrees at Northwestern and work primarily with preschool children here at _____."

In none of these examples did the individual provide a detailed resume; rather, each statement included the clinician's name and title and a brief notation of professional experience.

Opening an Information-Getting Interview

The opening or beginning phase of an interview to obtain information sets the tone and the stage for the conversations that follow. This phase can motivate interviewees to participate freely and communicate effectively and accurately—or it can hinder an interview early on by limiting free participation and subsequently can reduce the flow of information. According to Stewart and Cash (1994), opening an interview involves providing verbal orientations to interviewees and, at the same time, facilitating rapport between the participants.

Developing Rapport and Setting the Tone

As Chapter 2 indicates, rapport really means a harmonious relationship between the parties. The development and maintenance of rapport are important at all times during interviewing and counseling sessions. Ivey (1994) comments that rapport is important because, "unless the client has some liking for you, you won't go very far" (p. 152). Rapport is expedited by clinician punctuality; an attractive and comfortable setting; and clients knowing, at least in general terms, what to expect during the interview and from the relationship.

Rapport also is assisted by a host of other interviewer characteristics, and verbal and nonverbal communicative skills, addressed in Chapters 2 through 4. It is also assisted by cultural sensitivity and knowledge when working with clients from other cultures (see Chapter 8).

Initial comments during the opening of the interview orient interviewees by defining the participants' roles and indicating some of the activities that will follow. The tone of the interview is affected here by the attitudes an interviewer projects. Peterson and Marquardt (1994) note that clinicians and clients are not on "equal ground." Rather, interviewees typically have come to clinicians for help and direction, so clients expect that most of the questions and direction will come from the interviewer (Shipley & Wood, 1996).

The opening phase is structured as clinicians introduce (or reintroduce) themselves, briefly describe their role, and convey the purposes of a meeting. Clinicians should not assume that clients understand the specific purposes of an interview or the nature of the information that may be requested (Peterson & Marquardt, 1994). Effective interviewers describe in general terms what will be expected from interviewees and any limitations to the services that will be provided. During this orientation phase, it is also helpful to tell clients how any information obtained will be used, why the information is needed, and to whom it may be revealed. Finally, it is a good idea to remind clients how much time an interview is expected to take.

As Donaghy (1990) states, the beginning of the opening phase may include:

- An introduction or reintroduction of ourselves and reminding the other party of our role in the setting.
- An indication of any titles preferred.
- Any information that has been obtained from other persons, or any work or preparation already done.
- The degree of confidentiality to be maintained.
- The nature of the roles to be assumed.

It is worth remembering that many people have difficulty recalling names after just one or two meetings. Names that are unusual or difficult to pronounce present additional problems. A business card, a name tag, or a conspicuously placed desk plate can help people remember names. Knowledge of the clinician's role in the setting (e.g., clinical supervisor, speech-language pathologist, audiologist, intern, student teacher) prevents confusion so clients are less likely to make erroneous assumptions about the interviewer's authority or capacities. Regarding personal titles, it can be embarrassing for clients to discover that they have referred to an interviewer as Mr. or Ms. when Dr. would have been more appropriate. Embarrassment or even feelings of disillusionment or betrayal sometimes occur when patients learn interviewers whom they have called Dr. do not hold such a degree.

The following illustrates what a clinician might say when meeting a couple for the first time in a private waiting area:

> "Mr. and Mrs. Wallace, I am Ms. Sandoval, one of the speech-language pathologists at the center. I will be evaluating John's speech today. Before I see him, I'd like to spend a few minutes with both of you to get an idea of the things you are noticing about his speech. Once we've finished, I will see John by himself and later we'll talk about some of the things I've found. Please follow me to my office."

Once the clinician and couple have arrived in an office or conference area, it is appropriate to reiterate and expand on some of the general points made just moments earlier.

> "Again, my name is Ms. Sandoval and I am a speech-language pathologist. I'd like to spend the next few minutes getting your impressions of your son's speech. Then I'll see John and evaluate his speech. After that, we'll talk again. I'll share my findings and impressions with you at that time. The entire process should take about an hour and a half."

These examples help illustrate how a brief and succinct opening phase can serve to orient the party being interviewed. An opening orientation should, of course, be modified according to any particular setting or clinical needs. Some period of brief chit-chat may be useful with some interviewees, particularly those from diverse backgrounds. This can be done at the beginning of the opening phase.

Transition from the Opening to the Body of the Interview

The opening phase of the interview is usually brief, but it alerts people about what to expect. It also sets the stage for the body of the interview. During the body of the interview, clinicians focus on understanding the client, reviewing any appropriate histories necessary (medical, developmental speech, educational, and so forth), and discussing a client's perceptions of any communicative difficulties being experienced. The actual transition between the opening phase and body of the interview occurs when the first piece of information about a client is solicited; for example:

"Tell me about what brought you here today."

"I'm interested in learning more about your (or your child's, your spouse's, your parent's) speech. Tell me about some of your concerns."

Donaghy (1990) comments:

> *The opening question would encourage interviewees to give information. It should be nonthreatening and request information which the interviewee can easily answer. Usually, the opening question is quite general because general questions are less stressful and help interviewees relax. They allow respondents to ease into the body of the interview. The opening question should assume consent on the part of the interviewee—you should use positive phrasing such as, "Suppose you tell me about _____" rather than, "I wonder if you would tell me _____." (p. 92)*

The first few words and thoughts an interviewer expresses can be particularly significant in that they often reveal focuses and degrees of concern very early in an interview (Donaghy, 1990; Garrett, 1982). Several examples of initial statements from parents, with possible interpretations of the concerns expressed, illustrate these points.

"John's speech is very unclear and he's withdrawing from everyone. We hate to see this happen. It's killing us inside to see him just clam up." (There is a high level of concern, a focus on the child's emotional reactions, and another potential focus on the parents' reactions.)

"He can't make several sounds yet and we're afraid this may affect him when he starts to read. You know how once kids get behind in reading it seems like they never catch up." (Potentially a little less concern than the first example, with a focus on future academic abilities.)

"I had a cousin who stuttered real bad and we just want to make sure that Julia is not developing this type of problem." (Concern is present, but we are not yet quite sure of the level or focus of that concern other than stuttering having occurred within the family.)

"Jennifer's speech is OK but the doctor insisted that we come see you anyway." (Parent does not appear real concerned. This person may be following through out of politeness to someone else or was "coerced" into it. It is also possible that more concern will come out later.)

In these examples, there are very different focuses of concern (from "clamming up" to learning to read) and degrees of concern (from "it's killing us inside" to no apparent concern) being expressed. Interviewers should make a mental note, then add to or modify these impressions throughout the session.

In addition to information about levels and focuses of concern, interviewees' beginning statements can help provide insight into clients' educational background or overall insight into a problem. For example, someone who expresses concern about their child's sibilant distortions may have a considerably different amount of information than someone who just knows their child "talks funny." During clients' statements of the problem, clinicians listen for information concerning what clients think the difficulties are, their feelings about potential causes of the problem, and the ways they have tried to resolve the problem.

Getting started can be difficult for some interviewees. In such cases, it is helpful to start by noting briefly that it can be difficult to know where to begin (Benjamin, 1981). An interviewer might help with a comment like, "I know it can be difficult to know where to begin, but I need to know about your voice and the problems you are having." When a client has difficulty with a statement of the problem, the clinician should take care to phrase an open question that is neither too ambiguous nor too specific: "Tell me a little about your speech problem." How an interviewee responds will then determine how the interviewer should continue. By phrasing the opening question in an open-ended manner, clinicians avoid inhibiting or restricting clients. This can be particularly useful with some individuals from diverse backgrounds.

In the event of more extreme problems getting started, it is sometimes helpful to employ a series of closed question to get the person moving. However, these closed questions should not be in particularly sensitive or emotion-laden areas. Open questions are then asked once the patient has started opening up.

Important clues about interviewees' attitudes toward an interview situation or even toward the interviewer may be revealed (Garrett, 1982). These feelings may include ambivalence, confusion, fear, or even hostility. For example, patients sometimes tell clinicians "I don't need to be here but _____ is making me," inquire immediately if Dr. _____ is really any good, seek reaffirmation that nothing in the session will hurt, and so forth. An indication of hostility or anger in a client's opening statement may warrant a quick change in approach—or at least alert the interviewer to problems that may need to be addressed further.

Body of the Information-Getting Interview

It is during the body of the information-getting interview that an interviewer gains potentially important information about the client, including information about the development and present status of the client's communicative skills and appropriate medical, educational, therapeutic, and social histories (Peterson & Marquardt, 1994). Discussion often includes items of particular significance from the written case history form. In the following sections, the sequence of the interview is considered first; this is followed by some of the content applicable to the body of many information-getting interviews.

Sequence of the Body

The different types of open and closed questions, and primary and secondary questions, were described in Chapter 4. The general sequences of interviews also were discussed in that chapter. The two discussed were the *funnel sequence* and the *inverted funnel sequence* (Stewart & Cash, 1994). Recall that a funnel sequence moves from open to closed questions, from primary to secondary questions. This allows interviewers to move from more general to more specific types of information. A funnel sequence is useful when obtaining information in initial interviews. Clinicians begin by asking an open question about a topic, then narrow down a topic into specific details relating to that area. Different sub-areas of discussion can also be addressed in this manner. An open question is used first and closed questions then help generate the information needed in that sub-area. When the topic has been discussed adequately, an open question is then used to introduce the next sub-area of discussion ("You also mentioned concern about hearing"). Obviously, closed secondary questions then allow more extensive discussion of this topic before moving on to the next subject.

The inverted-funnel approach (closed to open) is less useful for most information-getting interviews, but it can be helpful in some instances. An inverted funnel can be used when working with some reluctant clients who are reticent to share their real feelings and with patients who are not talking much. This sequence also is helpful with some clients who may not feel there is a problem, or with others who are unsure what the problems really are. By asking questions requiring specific types of information first, inroads are sometimes made as these clients begin to see that there really is some reason for concern, or the potential areas of difficulty.

Content of the Body

The major items that have been noted on a written case history are often discussed and considered in detail during the body of the interview. Many of these items are found on the case history forms in Appendices A, B, and C at the back of this book. Most diagnoses, estimates of prognosis, and initial plans for remediation or treatment result from at least two sources, and often three. These are the information-getting interview, any diagnostic/assessment testing and observations performed and, when available and appropriate, information from other professionals involved with the case.

Some of the topics that are discussed in many information-getting interviews are presented in the following sections. However, the types of information that would allow clinicians to make a diagnosis are beyond the scope of this book and are not considered here. For more specific information regarding diagnostic and assessment procedures, the reader should consult other texts dealing specifically with diagnostic procedures (e.g., Haynes et al., 1992; Hutchinson, Hanson, & Mecham, 1979; Meitus & Weinberg, 1983; Nation & Aram, 1991; Peterson & Marquardt, 1994; Shipley & McAfee, 1992; Tomblin, Morris, & Spriestersbach, 1994), or resources dealing with specific types of communicative disorders. Assessment information pertaining specifically to clients from linguistically and culturally diverse populations is available in resources such as Cheng (1991), Hamayan and Damico (1991), Langdon (1992), Mattes and Omark (1991), and Roseberry-McKibbin (1995).

Identifying information.   A clinician may need to confirm data identifying the patient, such as addresses, telephone numbers, any third-party payers (e.g., public or private insurance), and so forth. This information can be important for adequate recordkeeping purposes. Although important, there can be risks when clinicians focus too much attention or time on these areas. Some clients may feel that a clinician is more concerned with "business matters" than with the communicative problems at hand. Clinicians should avoid becoming overly involved with these procedural details and losing valuable time and focus.

Family histories.   A number of disorders (e.g., stuttering, hearing loss, mental impairment, certain genetic syndromes) tend to run in families. Clinicians may need to try to determine any possible environmental or genetic links that may be related to diagnosis and subsequent treatment (see Gerber, 1990, or Jung, 1989). Clinicians should also determine how family members react and feel about the communicative problem. Many times the presence of anxiety can be a motivating factor for clients, parents, or other caregivers. At other times, the presence of anxiety can be counterproductive; alert clinicians should be able to detect such anxiety and estimate its effects.

When asking about family history, clinicians need to ask about the ages of family members; about educational history; about occupational history; and about past or present speech and language difficulties of parents, siblings, or relatives. If other family members also have or had communicative difficulties, it may be important for a clinician to obtain a history of the problems and any treatment received. It may be helpful for the clinician to inquire about where, how, by whom, and for how long family members were treated, and about the results of the treatment.

Attitudes toward a communicative disorder may be affected by a person's or caregiver's past experience with such a problem. For example, parents in a family that has a history of stuttering may experience considerable anxiety about their youngster who is beginning to stutter. On the other hand, parents in a family with a history of mild articulation problems that have been outgrown may not be too concerned about their child's inability to produce certain sounds well.

Familial attitudes can be influenced by cultural factors. For example, in the Southeast Asian Hmong community, physical or obvious mental disorders are taken more seriously than other difficulties (Hegde & Davis, 1995). Many Asians feel that handicapping conditions are those that are "visible." Other problems may be thought to result from "not trying hard enough" (Bebout & Arthur, 1992). Some Hispanic families also have more difficulties accepting less visible disabilities.

Developmental and motor histories.   When clinicians are treating communicative disorders in children and adolescents, it may be important to become knowledgeable about a client's prenatal, natal, and postnatal histories. Having this knowledge can aid in determining a diagnosis and, sometimes, in the isolation of an etiology. Specifically, clinicians may need to learn the length of the pregnancy, any illnesses a mother suffered during pregnancy, the child's birth weight, any physical anomalies or dysfunctions identified at birth, and so forth. It is sometimes imperative that clients or clients' parents or other caregivers understand why each question is being asked in any of these areas. Thus, it is sometimes necessary for clinicians to offer a rationale for asking certain questions.

Information about motor development is important because speech is a motor function. Problems with muscle tone, coordination, or symmetry may direct an examiner toward specific areas of the communicative mechanism. Clinicians may be concerned with problems, such as hypertonicity or hypotonicity, or difficulties with sitting, standing, and walking. Feeding problems, particularly those involving chewing, sucking, and swallowing, may be discussed in detail. Other pertinent areas may include tongue movement, weight gain, and independence of and adequacy in feeding. Data pertaining to these motor development milestones provide a reference base for examiners who will eventually make judgments about the adequacy of the speech mechanism. Physical concerns that require a medical referral can also be revealed when motor development is discussed.

Educational and social background.   An educational history is not absolutely necessary with every client, but it is usually helpful with most children. In some cases, it provides valuable insight into a child's intellectual potential, social maturity, expectations of parents and others, and the consistency of the client's performance across settings (Peterson & Marquardt, 1990). There are some instances when school performance is related to the presence of a communicative disorder. For example, a child may refuse to participate in verbal tasks because of a speech problem and, therefore, do poorly in those activities. Another child with a language deficiency may have difficulty learning academic subjects. Still another child who does not seem to be paying attention may have a hearing loss, attention deficit disorder, or another learning problem. Some children, particularly those who have immigrated recently, may not be in school, may have started school only recently, or may have attended a number of schools in different locations.

In the affective domain, some clients may become aggressive while others withdraw because peers have mocked or teased them about their speech. Of course, many other examples of problems in educational and interactional history, which relate in some way to a communicative disorder, could be given.

Socioeconomic background. As Peterson and Marquardt (1994) comment:

> *Socioeconomic classification systems may have a number of variables in their formulae, but most commonly include source (rather than amount) of income, occupation, and education of the parents.... The purpose in gathering social, cultural, and economic information is to help you determine cultural influences or opportunities available to the child [or adult].* (p. 39)

Social, cultural, and socioeconomic information can be important because it may reveal influences and conditions that impinge on the opportunities available for a client. The background or culture of certain children or adults may also influence the ways in which clinicians need to interact with those clients, affect the alternatives for service available, or influence some of the clinician's suggestions for speech stimulation or treatment.

Speech and language histories. Speech, language, and hearing development and skills are of primary concern to professionals in communicative disorders. Therefore, there will be considerable emphasis within this area during most pre-assessment interviews. The histories taken, and thus the questions asked, vary according to the type of client and communicative difficulty being seen. For example, more speech and language development information is needed for children than for adults. The focus of questions also differs when seeing different types of disorders—the production of specific sounds, sound-production patterns, and intelligibility is of greater concern with articulation cases than with many voice cases. Questions about chewing, sucking, and swallowing are necessary with dysphagia, but may not be asked with certain fluency problems, and so forth. The point is that the focus of attention is dictated by different combinations of the disorder seen, age, and cultural influences.

With children, questions may be asked about various speech and language development milestones, including ages and stages at which different language skills developed. The pragmatic use of language is also important. Realizing the inherent limitations of normative data, and the variability with which children learn and use language, such information still enables clinicians to compare speech and language skills with "normal expectations." Clinicians can also determine how caregivers feel about the child's rate and sequence of speech and language development, what expectations they have in mind, and what their aspirations and expectations are (Peterson & Marquardt, 1994). It is important, therefore, for clinicians to have a good background in speech and language development so that they can understand and interpret case history information and clinical observations. However, careful clinicians also are aware that norms differ across cultural groups, so they do not inappropriately generalize information from known norms to individuals with whom certain data is inapplicable.

It may not be possible or even necessary to obtain detailed prenatal, birth, or developmental histories for most adults. Rather, their recent medical histories are often most pertinent. However, historical factors that might be considered in certain cases include childhood or adulthood diseases, injuries, hospitalizations, surgeries, and medications.

In some cases, physiological or medical information may be necessary to help clinicians determine a diagnosis. Such information may clarify the nature of a specific communicative disorder and help the clinician determine a client's needs and possibilities for improvement. For example, the diagnosis of acquired aphasia requires observation of a variety of speech and language behaviors across several modalities to collect evidence of organic damage to the brain. Professionals sometimes observe regression or deterioration of speech, language, or hearing abilities in patients with medical problems; clinicians who are alert for such changes in patients' communicative behaviors become critical monitors for physicians and patients themselves.

As alluded to earlier, there are a number of questions that can be asked about any particular disorder type. Shipley and McAfee (1992) list a number of questions that may be appropriate within the traditionally viewed, general speech and language categories (see Appendix 5-A). These are not intended as a checklist of questions to be asked. They should not be used for "question-and-answer" interviews, but rather, as topics and possible questions that can be modified for each particular client. Also notice that follow-up questions would be needed, depending on particular responses to many of the questions.

Special case histories.   Most information-getting interviews will at least touch on the general topics noted in the previous sections and/or in Appendix 5-A. More specific questions are often necessary depending on the type of communicative disorder. For example, with aphasia, Darley (1978) emphasizes gathering information about the following:

- *The patient's premorbid and present abilities,*
- *Personality characteristics and subsequent changes in the patient's personality,*

- *The patient's past interests and occupation,*
- *The patient's educational background,*
- *The patient's environment and those who will best facilitate progress in the environment,*
- *Associated sensory and motor disturbances, and*
- *Deterioration in other cognitive functions.* (p. 91)

Specific types of information are also necessary with other disorders: closed-head injury, dysphagia, laryngectomy, traumatic brain injury, and so forth. A sample case history for voice is in Appendix B at the back of this book.

Multicultural histories. Chapter 8 includes a discussion of a number of factors related to cross-cultural practice. Clinicians are also encouraged to read about other cultures and to perform ethnographic interviews. An ethnographic interview is essentially an interview with members of the culture from which their clients come (see Lund & Duchan, 1993; Mattes & Omark, 1991; Roseberry-McKibbin, 1995; Westby, 1990; or others). These interviews help clinicians get a perspective of the other culture and provide important information about cultural attitudes, traditions, and values. Such factors as educational values, views of handicapping conditions, decision-making processes, attitudes toward receiving outside help, expressions of courtesy or respect, and many other factors can be learned. Cheng's (1991) "Background Information Questionnaire" was developed specifically for use with clients from diverse backgrounds (see Appendix C).

Important Areas to Address Across Different Disorders

Irrespective of the type of communicative difficulty being assessed, there are some rather universally applicable questions that often need to be asked. These questions are discussed in the following sections.

When and how did the problem develop? This question identifies when a difficulty began to emerge, and how it has progressed. With certain disorders, such as stuttering in early childhood, some clinicians use this information to assist in the diagnosis and recommendations for treatment (McFarlane, Fujiki, & Brinton, 1984). The course of certain disorders, whether they are sudden or gradual, may have implications for organic etiology that require medical investigation. A diagnosis may also be based, at least in part, on the course and history of the disorder. For example, many aphasias are sudden and episode-specific, while the course of disorders associated with Parkinson or Alzheimer's syndromes is progressive.

Has the problem changed since it was first noticed? Has the problem gotten better, worse, or is it about the same? Depending on the type of communicative difficulty being exhibited, the answers to such questions influence clinical impressions and recommendations. For example, a clinician may not recommend treatment for a child with one or two minor articulation errors who seems to be improving "week by week." The recommendation might be considerably different if a child were not improving, or if the difficulty were becoming more pronounced.

The negative progression of communicative symptoms can signal the need for speech-language pathology services, audiologic intervention, medical referral, psychological referral, or educational consultation. This point deserves to be emphasized because communicative skills do not deteriorate without some physical, emotional, or environmental cause.

Are there times when the problem varies, or circumstances that create fluctuations in the difficulties? The communicative behaviors associated with many speech and hearing disorders are relatively stable. However, factors related to a particular problem may vary according to the type of problem and/or various environmental conditions. Understanding sources of variability can help clinicians establish a diagnosis but, more often, this helps determine treatment focuses and treatment recommendations. The following examples help illustrate the point: (1) Treatment efforts might focus on telephone work for someone who was dysfluent primarily on the telephone. (2) If a client were dysfluent primarily in the presence of certain individuals, those persons might need to be included in treatment efforts. (3) The teacher who experienced dysphonia only when teaching, or whose voice became progressively worse only on days of teaching, would seem to need specific attention on the use of a better voice when teaching.

How does the client react to the communicative problem? How do parents or other caregivers react to the problem? Answers to such questions provide insight into how much a communicative disorder is affecting the people involved. Sometimes, there will be only minimal impact. At other times, even a minor problem can have a considerable impact on individuals who are affected. The answers also reveal how much a client may be "hurting" and what a client's or caregiver's motivation may be for wanting help.

Sometimes, a client may have little concern about a problem despite the fact that significant others are deeply concerned. Sometimes, a patient may be deeply affected by a communicative problem while others in the environment do not share this degree of concern. There are also instances when a person's concern for a child or other family member is actually helping perpetuate a difficulty. All of these cases, and a number of other possibilities, yield important implications for determining how to approach and serve patients.

Where else has the interviewee (or the interviewee's child or other family member) been seen? What did other professionals find or suggest? It is not unusual for written case histories to provide space for respondents to indicate where other evaluations have been sought, but the results of these evaluations may or may not be available to the clinician. It is useful to determine where other evaluations or treatment services have been secured and how a patient perceived these services.

Such information provides clinicians with insight into how individuals feel about the other professional settings, what types of treatment were received in those settings, the general effectiveness of such treatment, and how a client feels about treatment in general. Asking these questions also helps clinicians avoid being caught off guard if a client informs them later that their results, conclusions, or recommendations differ from those of professionals seen previously.

Such questions also prepare clinicians for future discussions with the client, such as during information-giving interviews following assessment sessions. This is particularly important when clinician's findings or treatment methods differ from what a patient has experienced previously. The intention here is not to "second guess" or otherwise undermine the credibility of other persons or agencies; rather, it is to understand that differences exist among various service providers. Discussion of such differences may be needed with certain clients.

Asking where else a client has been seen also helps clinicians detect clients who are "shopping" for answers that fit into their beliefs. Mowrer (1988) points out that some clients seek services or opinions that will conform with their own ideas regarding whether a problem exists. The possibility that a client is shopping for an answer that agrees with a personal viewpoint is sometimes revealed when clinicians ask about previous services. Clinicians should also recognize that shopping sometimes occurs because of ineffective communication between clients and professionals (Leigh & Marshall, 1983).

Service sources other than speech and hearing personnel may have also been consulted. These other sources could include astrologers, clergy, former teachers, or others. Some clients from certain ethnic backgrounds may have consulted some form of a healer or spiritualist (Chan, 1992b; Roseberry-McKibbin, 1995; Zuniga, 1992).

How has the interviewee tried to help? The answer to this question provides interviewers with insight into a patient's communicative difficulties and also into what patients or caregivers have tried to do to assist with the problems. It is important to realize that whether or not they have employed the best possible solution, most people have tried to help with good intentions. For example, a parent who consistently tells a child who is stuttering to "stop, take a deep breath, think about what you want to say, then talk without making all those ba-ba-ba's," may be doing so with good intentions. This realization allows a clinician to look at the *what* rather than focusing solely on the *why* of some action. It is not unusual for human beings to do the wrong things for the right reasons!

Knowing what has already been done provides clinicians with insight into what should now be done. Often clinicians encourage caregivers who are providing the right types of help to continue with such activities. At other times, only minor instruction is required to help someone who is attempting to do the right things become more effective. However, there are also instances when clinicians need to help clients or caregivers alter activities that are counterproductive to improving communicative abilities. In such cases, some form of instruction or counseling may be necessary. The important point is that clinicians must be aware of what is occurring in the environment. This awareness provides a basis on which to begin shaping future recommendations or attempts to modify existing attitudes or behaviors.

Culture plays a large role here as we modify what are essentially belief systems or traditional ways of doing something. For example, Maestas and Erickson (1992) comment that

> *trying to change the values and beliefs of parents may result in undermining their self-confidence and destroying their self-esteem. Instead, working within the framework of their culture may promote trust and confidence in often otherwise reluctant clients. Elements of the client's culture can be incorporated into a therapy program without abandoning or compromising the communication specialist's original remedial plan.... Professionals acknowledging and respecting these traditional beliefs may help clients cooperate more fully with their therapy programs.* (p. 9)

Can the interviewee describe the specific communicative difficulty? Or, can the interviewee imitate the problem? Responses to these questions often provide clinicians with considerable insight into interviewees' perceptions of the problem at hand, and the degree of specificity with which the interviewee has tried to evaluate and understand the difficulty. For example, parents who report that their child substitutes *w* for *r* and *f* for *th* are exhibiting considerably more knowledge and insight than those who only can describe the child's same speech pattern as sounding "babyish." The specificity of knowledge about the sound errors is very different in these two cases. Clinicians need to understand such factors in order to approach future discussions appropriately.

Has the client been seen by an appropriate specialist? Clinicians need to know if a patient has consulted other specialists. Many times, the voice case or the hearing aid candidate needs to be evaluated by an otolaryngologist; the neurologically involved patient by a neurologist; the emotionally disturbed person by a psychologist, another type of mental health-care provider, or a special educator; the mentally handi-capped child by a psychologist or special educator; the person with severe dental problems by a dentist or orthodontist; and so forth. Clinicians may need information from other specialists and should not be afraid to ask about such matters. Again, this information helps clinicians make needed assessments and develop future recommendations.

Closing the Interview

The body of an information-getting interview is concluded when a clinician has finished obtaining necessary information about the client, the client's history, and any other pertinent details deemed necessary to understand the case. The clinician then moves to the last phase of the interview.

The closing segment of the information-getting interview is relatively brief and concise. Major features of a closing are (1) providing a summary of what has been discussed; (2) giving interviewees opportunities to add on any information gained, or clarify any interviewer misperceptions; (3) expressing appreciation to the other party; and (4) revealing the next steps in the process.

Interviewers begin by summarizing the major information that has been obtained. This helps the clinician demonstrate to clients that they have been heard and understood. It also gives those who have been interviewed an opportunity to identify any information that requires clarification, expansion, or correction. Once all information has been summarized, and corrected or added to if necessary, clinicians express appreciation for the interviewee's efforts: "I appreciate the information you have provided. It should be helpful in understanding your speech (or your son's speech, your mother's speech)." Finally, the clinician closes the interview by revealing the next steps that will occur. The actual closing statement is sometimes rather general, but provides enough information so that clients know what will be done next.

> "Now I would like to spend some time with your son. I will listen to his speech in several contexts and evaluate the speech difficulty. That should take about an hour. After I finish, we'll talk again and I will share my findings and recommendations with you. Thank you again for your help."

The same model is useful when the person interviewed is also the patient.

> "Now let's turn our attention to assessing your dysfluencies and whether we can improve your speech. I'm going to have you read some materials and then we'll check your hearing. I'll let you know what I'm finding as we are going along. We'll also spend a few minutes at the end to discuss what I have found and what we should do next."

Concluding Comments

Professionals working with communicative disorders are routinely involved in obtaining a number of different types of information in their diagnostic and therapeutic interactions. With first-time patients and families, an information-getting interview should be preceded by appropriate presession orientation for interviewees. The actual interview proceeds through three distinct phases—the opening phase, the body, and the closing. Interviewers orient interviewees toward what will occur during the opening phase, while simultaneously helping build rapport. A transition is made from the opening phase to the body of the interview when interviewees provide the first substantial piece of information about the case. During the body of the interview, interviewers gain the information needed about a client and the client's communicative difficulty, including background information about speech, language, and hearing or other appropriate histories. Then, in the closing phase, clinicians summarize what has been said, allow clients to clarify any misconceptions and add anything needed, express appreciation to the interviewee, and direct or orient interviewees toward the activities or interactions that will follow.

The opening and closing phases of information-getting interviews are rather short and succinct; the body of the interview is much longer and is really the "meat" of the interview. Successful information-getting interviews result in an adequate depth and scope of information that, when combined with information from an actual diagnostic session, will provide an excellent overall picture of the communicative problem and its various ramifications.

Interviews to obtain information are also conducted when someone is enrolled for ongoing treatment; for example, to gain information about some testing (medical, educational, psychological) done elsewhere, to find out if certain communicative behaviors are generalizing outside the clinical or educational environment, to learn more regarding how someone is feeling about a client's progress, and so forth. These interviews use the same basic structure, including opening, body, and closing phases. The content of the body is about rather specific topics, compared to a large body of potential information during assessment-related interviewing.

APPENDIX 5-A

COMMONLY ASKED TYPES OF QUESTIONS

The following types of questions are commonly asked in many information-getting, or case history, interviews. Be aware that asking every question is not necessary or even appropriate with all clients. Do not use the questions as an interviewing checklist; rather, select appropriate questions and adapt as needed to help gain a more complete understanding of a client's problems. When questioning a parent or caregiver about a child, substitute the words "your child" or use the child's name for "you" or "your."

Articulation

Describe your concerns about your speech.

What is your native language? What language do you speak often?

What language is spoken most often at home? At school? At work?

How long have you been concerned about your speech? Who first noticed the problem?

Describe your speech when the problem was first noticed. Has it improved over time?

What do you think is the cause of your speech problem?

What sounds are most difficult for you?

Is it difficult for you to repeat what other people have said?

Are there times when your speech is better than others?

How well does your family understand you? Do they ask you to repeat yourself?

How well do your friends and acquaintances understand you? Do they ask you to repeat yourself?

Does your speech affect your interactions with other people?

How does it affect your work? Your social activities? Your school activities?

What have you done to try to improve your speech?

Have you had speech therapy before? When? Where? With whom? What were the results?

During the time you have been with me, has your speech been typical? Is it better or worse than usual?

Source: From Kenneth G. Shipley and Julie G. McAfee, *Assessment in Speech-Language Pathology: A Resource Manual* (pp. 7-10). Copyright 1992 by and reprinted with the permission of Singular Publishing Group, San Diego, CA.

Language (Child)

Use the child's name rather than "your child" whenever possible.

Describe your concerns about your child's language.

What is your child's native language? What language does your child speak most often?

What language is spoken most often at home? At school? At work?

Who does your child interact with most often? What kind of activities do they do together?

Does your child seem to understand you? Others?

How well do you understand your child?

Does your child maintain eye contact?

How does your child get your attention (through gestures, verbalizations, etc.)?

How does your child express needs and wants?

Approximately how many words does your child understand?

Approximately how many words does your child use?

Provide an estimate of your child's average sentence length.

Approximately how many words does your child use in his (or her) longest sentences?

Does your child follow

    Simple commands (e.g., put that away)?

    Two-part commands (e.g., get your shoes and brush your hair)?

    Three-part commands (e.g., pick up your toys, brush your teeth, and get in bed)?

Does your child ask questions?

Does your child use:

    Nouns (e.g., boy, car)?

    Verbs (e.g., jump, eat)?

    Adjectives (e.g., big, funny)?

    Adverbs (e.g., quickly, slowly)?

    Pronouns (e.g., he, they)?

    Conjunctions (e.g., and, but)?

    -ing endings (e.g., going, jumping)?

    Past-tense word forms (e.g., went, jumped)?

    Plurals (e.g., dogs, toys)?

    Possessives (e.g., my mom's, the dog's)?

    Comparatives (e.g., slower, bigger)?

Does your child appear to understand cause-and-effect relationships? The function of objects?

Is your child able to imitate immediately? Following a short lapse of time? How accurate is the imitation?

Can your child narrate or talk about experiences?

Does your child know how to take turns in conversation?

Is your child's speech usually appropriate to the situation?

Does your child participate in symbolic play (e.g., use of a stick to represent a microphone)?

Language (Adult)

What is your native language? What language do you speak most often?

Do you have a problem in your native language and in English?

How long have you been concerned about your language? Who first noticed the problem?

Describe your language abilities when the problem was first noticed. Has it improved over time?

Do you read? How often? What kinds of books do you read?

Describe your education. Did you have any problems learning?

What do you think is the cause of your language problem?

What does your family think about the problem?

Does your language affect your interaction with other people? How does it affect your work? Your social activities?

Have you had any accidents or illnesses that have affected your language?

What have you done to try to improve your language skills?

Have you had language therapy before? When? Where? With whom? What were the results?

Stuttering

Describe your concerns about your speech.

When did you first begin to stutter? Who noticed it? In what type of speaking situations did you first notice it?

Describe your stuttering when it was first noticed. How has it changed over time?

Did anyone else in the family stutter (parents, brothers, sisters, grandparents, uncles, aunts, cousins, etc.)?

Do they still stutter? Did they have therapy? If so, did it help?

Why do you think you stutter?

Does the stuttering bother you? How?

How does your family react to the problem?

How do your friends and acquaintances react to the problem?

What do you do when you stutter?

When you stutter, what do you do to try to stop it? Does your strategy work? If yes, why do you think it works? If no, why not?

In what situations do you stutter the most (over the telephone; speaking to a large group; speaking to your spouse, boss, or someone in a position of authority; etc.)?

In what situations do you stutter the least (speaking to a child, speaking to your spouse, etc.)?

Do you avoid certain speaking situations? Describe these.

Do you avoid certain sounds or words? Describe these.

Does your stuttering problem vary from day to day? How does it vary? Why do you think it varies?

What have you done to try to eliminate the stuttering (previous therapy, self-help books, etc.)? What were the results?

Have you had speech therapy before? When? Where? With whom? What were the results?

Does your stuttering give you difficulties at work, at school, or at home? Are there other places that it gives you trouble?

Have you had any illnesses or accidents that seemed to affect your speech? Describe these.

During the time you have been with me, has your speech been typical? Are you stuttering more or less than usual?

Voice

Describe your concerns about your voice?

How long have you had the voice problem? Who first noticed it?

Describe your voice when the problem was first noticed. How has it changed over time?

What do you think is the cause of your voice problem?

Do you speak a lot at work? At home? On the telephone? At social events or in large groups?

What types of activities are you involved in?

Do you ever run out of breath when you talk? Describe those situations.

In what speaking situations is your voice the worst? In what speaking situations is your voice the best?

Is your voice better or worse at different times of the day?

How does your family react to your voice problem?

How do your friends and acquaintances react to your voice?

How does your voice affect your interactions with other people? How does it affect your work? Your social activities? School?

What have you done to try to resolve the problem?

Have you seen an ear, nose, and throat specialist? What were the results?

Have you had speech therapy before? When? Where? With whom? What were the results?

Have you had any illnesses or accidents that seemed to affect your voice? Describe these.

During the time you have been with me, has your voice been typical? Is it better or worse than usual?

$$Chapter \quad 6$$

Providing Information

Imparting accurate, understandable information about clients and their communicative disorders is an important responsibility of clinicians in all settings. Sharing information often occurs after assessment sessions with children, and during or after many assessment sessions with adults. Information regarding treatment progress is, or should be, shared on an ongoing basis when someone is enrolled for ongoing services. There are also occasions when information is shared with others who are involved with the case—teachers, physicians, mental health professionals, and others (Mowrer, 1988). Of course, this is done with the client's or caregiver's permission. The importance of providing accurate and appropriate information cannot be understated—it is a very important professional responsibility.

Cunningham and Davis (1985) relate that the most frequent complaint cited by parents of special-needs children concern unsatisfactory communication with professionals. Too often, professionals provide insufficient, inaccurate, or even excessive information. This also occurs within communicative disorders and it causes some real problems for individuals needing services (Luterman, 1991; Martin, 1994). Haynes, Pindzola, and Emerick (1992) suggest that the most common complaint of patients in hospital and clinic settings is that they have not been kept well-informed of their conditions or progress. Referring to parents, Haynes et al. comment:

> *When not correctly informed, parents become misinformed and this leads to confusion, misunderstanding, and further compounding of the problem. It is our responsibility, therefore, to provide*

101

accurate, unemotional, objective information on the status of the individual's speech and hearing problem. (p. 46)

Often clinicians are not fully understood because of ineffective presentation technique or the inappropriate use of technical language. When confusion or misunderstanding occurs, relations between clinicians and clients or their caregivers suffer and rapport is undermined.

A clinician's effectiveness in providing information is related to the various factors discussed in the preceding chapters. Especially important are the enabling conditions—sensitivity, respect, empathy, objectivity, listening skills, motivation, and rapport—discussed in Chapter 2 and the ability to communicate effectively. Knowing what to share, when to share it, and how to share it are very important.

Conveying Information

Information is typically provided in person, although there are a few instances when this occurs by phone or correspondence. These exceptions are usually with other professionals rather than with clients or their caregivers. In the following sections, conveying information is discussed primarily in the context of a post-assessment interview. However, the same principles apply to other circumstances, such as providing information during an assessment session with adults or providing information about progress in therapy. These principles are simply modified as appropriate for other circumstances.

Like information-getting interviews (discussed in Chapter 5), an information-giving interview usually proceeds through three stages, or phases: (1) an opening, (2) the body, and (3) a distinct closing. Before describing these phases, the always-important area of preparation needs to be considered.

Preparing to Give Information

Adequate preparation is needed before opening any interview (Reilly, 1988; Shipley & Wood, 1996), and it is particularly important for an information-giving interview. An interview room should be free from clutter, appear professional, and be arranged appropriately for a serious discussion. Confidential materials, patients' folders, or any other materials that could violate someone else's confidentiality or be distracting, should be removed from sight. Appropriately sized chairs should be available for everyone involved. This is of particular concern in settings where clinicians also work with children in the same room.

If a client has been evaluated during a diagnostic session, it is important to allow adequate time for any materials to be collated, scored, and evaluated so that clinicians can share results from this information in the information-giving interview. When insufficient time is allowed, it is possible some information will not be available. It is also possible that rushing will result in scoring certain tests incorrectly, and basing certain assumptions on inaccurate information. Taking the time necessary for accurate, reliable test scoring and interpretation is important, particularly if some results could influence a clinician's judgment about the presence or extent of a problem.

For inexperienced and for experienced but cautious interviewers, it is helpful to list beforehand by general categories the major findings that need to be addressed in an information-giving interview. This listing helps clinicians develop an order for the interview, and it prevents inadvertently forgetting to share important information. However, clinicians should avoid relying on a checklist for each point and comment made during an interaction (Enelow & Swisher, 1986; Shipley & Wood, 1996). A "checklist interview" is often very noncommunicative and inflexible.

Opening the Interview

Most information-giving interviews are conducted separately from the diagnostic session, although many sessions include both, particularly with adults. When these are separate occasions, clinicians usually begin the interview with a brief, general orientation statement about what will be discussed.

> "I have evaluated your son's speech, and I want to share my findings and some suggestions with you."

> "Having talked with your physician and now evaluated your hearing, I'd like to share some of my findings and recommendations with you."

> "I finished evaluating Javier's language on Friday and talked with his teacher today. I'd like to share some of the information I have with you."

It is also helpful for the clinician to indicate approximately how much time will be involved and to report whether a satisfactory, representative sample of the client's communicative behavior was collected during the assessment session. A positive statement about how the client interacted or cooperated during the assessment can also be helpful, particularly with parents or with caregivers of "feisty" adults who were evaluated. Initial orientations that cover these topics are helpful because many interviewees are concerned about these areas, but sometimes do not mention this. Interviewees may be worried about certain time constraints—whether there will be enough time on the parking meter, whether there will be enough time to pick up another child, and so forth. Many interviewees, particularly parents, will be concerned about a child's behavior and if the communicative behavior of concern was exhibited during the diagnostic session. Such concerns, which frequently go unsaid, can affect an interviewee's concentration.

A clinician might open an information-giving interview with a statement such as the following:

> "Ben was very cooperative and worked hard during the whole session. I was able to get a good sample of his speech and how he's making his speech sounds. I want to take the next ten to fifteen minutes to share the results with you."

In this brief statement, the clinician describes the general behavior of the child, indicates that a good speech sample was obtained, notes the purpose of the interview, and suggests the approximate time anticipated for the discussion. Of course, the actual time may vary from the clinician's estimate, depending on the interviewee's needs. The same basic content areas apply to discussions of ongoing treatment; for example:

> "I have now seen your mother three times and she is working very hard. I'd like to talk about what we are doing and the progress I'm seeing. I also have some suggestions for use outside the clinic. Let's take about fifteen minutes and I'll share this with you."

This model can be adapted with different situations. Three different examples follow.

> "Maria was quite active during the session, but she did work hard on several tasks. I was able to get some of the information needed, but several things still need to be completed. I will need to see Maria again to finish the evaluation. Before scheduling her for another session, I do want to take about ten minutes to share several impressions with you."

> "Like many stroke victims, your father was very agitated and sometimes confused. But he cooperated with much of the testing and I have a pretty good idea of what needs to be done. In the next few minutes, I'd like to share some of my findings and suggestions with you."

> "Mrs. Knight, I know that some of the sounds you were listening for were difficult to hear and that it was hard to hear all the words I was saying. But you stayed with it and responded very consistently. Let's take the next few minutes and talk about your hearing."

These short statements follow the same model of describing a client's general behavior during the assessment session, the general adequacy of the behavior sampled, the time needed to discuss the findings, and the purpose of the present conversation. Impressions of a client's behavior that the orientation statement conveys should always be warranted by what actually took place; that is, do not say a client worked well if this is not the case. However, it is possible, in an objective and nonthreatening manner, to put positive and negative aspects of behavior in perspective. It is also true that we can find something positive in every individual (McFarlane, Fujiki, & Brinton, 1984).

> "Julia worked well the first five to ten minutes, then seemed to tire."
>
> "John was quite active, but I did get several things accomplished."
>
> "Jennifer was pretty upset at first, but she did eventually calm down. Once the crying subsided, I was able to _____ ."

The same general framework is used with reporting progress from ongoing treatment.

> "Jennifer had a few difficulties adjusting to what I was asking her to do the first two sessions, but she has now adjusted and is working hard. She seems to be enjoying our time together and is starting to progress in several areas. Let's take the next few minutes and I'll share some of what we are doing."

Statements of behavior that draw conclusions or that consist of a clinician's feelings about a client are unproductive. For example, statements, such as "He's really uncooperative!" or "She really behaved poorly," or questions—"Is he always like that?"—frequently do no more than engender negative feelings. Care also is necessary here with parents who might punish a child for "misbehaving." Some children may be punished, sometimes physically, for not cooperating fully or for not meeting a parent's expectations—and this is not our intention.

The opening of interviews to provide information is usually very short. Clinicians then move immediately into the most important part—the body of the interview.

Body of the Interview

Structure of the body.   The concepts of "funnel" and "inverted-funnel" sequences were introduced in Chapter 4 in relation to how open and closed questions are sequenced. These two sequences were discussed again in Chapter 5 as they apply to the sequencing of information sought in information-getting interviews. Recall that a funnel sequence starts with more open comments or questions before moving into more closed types of stimuli. An inverted-funnel sequence moves just the opposite, moving from closed to open. The same principles can apply to conveying information, particularly in post-assessment interviews. General, more overall or conclusive comments can be provided first, followed by more specific details or findings in a funnel sequence. Conversely, an inverted-funnel sequence involves providing more precise details or findings first, then moves to the more general information or overall conclusions. Both sequences are useful when conveying information to others.

It is helpful if, while preparing for an information-giving interview, clinicians try to judge how anxious an interviewee is about the communicative problem or any information that might be conveyed. Often, when an interviewee is highly anxious or highly concerned, it is best to share major conclusions (sometimes referred to as the "bottom line") at or near the beginning of the interview.

> "Mrs. Smith, John does have problems making a number of his speech sounds. He is going to need therapy to learn to make these sounds. The first thing I found was _____."

> "Mr. Richards, you do have a significant hearing loss and would benefit from a hearing aid. Here are some of the things I found _____."

Certain highly anxious clients will be so concerned about learning the major, or overall, conclusions that they are unable to effectively listen and process other information until they have heard those conclusions. A highly anxious student is often like this—hearing little of an instructor's feedback about the strengths or weaknesses of a given test or project because the real area of immediate concern, the bottom line, is the grade. For such students or such clients, sharing the bottom line (e.g., the grade) before providing specific feedback about *why* will allow opportunities for greater understanding of both the specific findings and any conclusions drawn.

Conversely, with less anxious and less concerned patients, or with individuals who have doubts regarding the existence or severity of a communicative difficulty, it is often helpful to present the more detailed, specific findings first (e.g., the specific results from a hearing test or the articulation testing) before sharing the overall or bottom-line conclusions. This order of presentation helps build a case for the conclusions offered and allows individuals to understand how any conclusions were reached. When clinicians build a case in this way, there is less chance that less anxious or doubting interviewees will reject the clinician's conclusions, either verbally or silently, before at least hearing all the details underpinning these conclusions.

Content of the interview.   Whether the bottom-line conclusions are presented at the beginning or at the end of the body of an interview, the major content includes the most important items that need to be shared. This typically includes information derived from an information-getting interview, observation, and any formal or informal testing performed.   Before beginning this type of interview, clinicians should determine the most salient points that they want interviewees to understand.

Clinicians overwhelm many interviewees with too much information too quickly, causing a lack of understanding and confusion (Luterman, 1991). Using a general guideline of three to five major points to share is helpful because clinicians are forced to identify and then convey the major points—and interviewees are allowed to focus on and truly understand these points. The three-to-five major points is a general rule; there may be only one or two major points in some interviews, or even six or seven in others. However, more than four or five important points is "stretching it" with many interactions. Of course, more than one or two points can stretch the limits with some clients, particularly with difficult-to-deal-with information, when a given interviewee does not comprehend what is being said, in the presence of language barriers, and so forth.

When clinicians present more than three to five major points, it is difficult for many patients to process them, let alone to recall them later. Sticking to a smaller number of points, and discussing anything else within the framework of those points, helps ensure that the most important points are discussed. Presenting more points often creates confusion regarding which points are really important and which are of secondary importance. Determining the major points to convey is relatively easy—list out the points that need to be shared and then rank order them in importance. Many times, clinicians find that some of the items they write out initially fall under certain other points listed. Some clinicians literally draw a line after the four or five most important points, saving items below the line for another occasion.

Using three to five major points is helpful even if a client's speech, language, or hearing skills are fine and there is no need for concern. In this case, the three to five major points might be positive findings having to do with normal speech–sound production, language, oral structure and function, and hearing.

It has been said that anything worth saying is worth saying at least three times. Haynes et al. (1992) suggest that clinicians need to, "repeat, repeat, repeat the important points—rephrasing each time" (p. 48). This is important when providing information because there is no guarantee that what is said will be heard or, more important, understood. Also, remember that people do not all process new information with equal speed or accuracy (Martin, 1994). When using planned repetitions, clinicians should vary their actual wordings each time a major thought is conveyed. Clinicians also need to remember that words alone do not always convey the full meaning of messages (Fenlason, 1962; Hutchinson, 1979; Roberts & Bouchard, 1989). Facial expression and other nonverbal behaviors are important parts of communicating information.

A majority of the information is provided by interviewees during information-*getting* interviews. With information-*giving* interviews, most of the information is provided by the clinician. However, when conducting an information-giving interview, clinicians can seek any additional clarifying information that is still needed from clients. Clinicians should also allow interviewees sufficient opportunities to seek any additional clarifying information they need or desire. The point is, interviews intended primarily to provide information are not "a one-way street."

Closing the Interview

Once the major points have been discussed and the clinician is confident that the other party has understood them, the interviewer moves into the closing phase. This phase allows the clinician to terminate the interaction systematically and smoothly. A good closing prevents the kind of awkward terminations that occur when "there doesn't seem to be anything else to talk about so we might as well stop." An appropriate closing consists of the following:

- Summarizing the main points discussed.
- Asking if there are any questions.
- Expressing appreciation for the interviewee's time, help, and interest.
- Sharing the next steps that will be taken.

Clinicians summarize the major points discussed, repeat any conclusions drawn, and reiterate the major suggestions or recommendations provided; for example:

> "I'm pleased we had this chance to talk. Again, our major findings were _____ . This is why I felt that _____ . What we need to consider doing next is _____ ."

This model allows clinicians to repeat the major findings and points of discussion, the conclusions, and the recommendations that have been shared in an easy-flowing, systematic manner. Often, the major points, which were determined prior to the interview, are the same items that end up being summarized in the closing phase. However, depending on what was actually discussed, there may be additional points that have now become important so these are also included in the final summary.

Opportunities to ask questions are provided throughout the body of the interview and, hopefully, clients will take advantage of this. In the closing, there is a final opportunity to seek additional information or clarification.

> "We've talked about a number of things. Let me stop for a moment. You probably have some additional questions about some of the things we've talked about."

> "We've talked about several aspects of your voice. If you had one or two questions you really wanted the answer to (or want me to go over again), what might they be?"

> "Is there something else you really wanted an answer to, or something that wasn't very clear?"

In some cases, particularly when difficult-to-deal-with information has been covered, interviewees need time to collect their thoughts and to think about the information conveyed. I sometimes recommend calling a "time-out" for this purpose.

> "There's something I need to grab from the next room. Why don't you think about anything we need to discuss further, or questions you still have. I'll be back in a minute or two and we'll discuss your questions."

This type of time-out allows clients to think about different areas discussed and then ask questions to clarify points that were not completely understood.

Another technique for stimulating questions is to tactfully ask some patients for a summary of the major points discussed; for example:

> "Suppose your wife (husband, parent, child, employer, physician, insurance company, one of my colleagues, etc.) were to ask you to talk about the most important things we discussed. What might you share?"

This request helps clinicians assess what information interviewees have and understand; it also allows the other party to discover areas that are still unclear. Thus, asking patients for this type of summary sometimes triggers clarifying questions.

Once all questions are satisfactorily addressed, clinicians thank those who were interviewed for their time, interest, or whatever else is appropriate. Any next steps in the clinical process are then briefly addressed. This can be as short as: "I'll be seeing Mark again Thursday, and you and I will talk again in about two weeks"; or it may be more detailed, depending on the circumstances.

Basic Principles of Human Nature and Sharing Information

Ten Principles of Human Nature

There are many variables that influence how people receive and react to information shared. A few of these include the interviewer's personality and communicative style, the types of information shared, how information is conveyed, and individual differences among those who are interviewed. Donaghy (1990, pp. 19-21) talks about ten basic principles of human nature that affect interactions. In the information that follows, the italicized comments are Donaghy's; the nonitalicized comments are adaptations of his thoughts.

1. *No two people are alike.* People do react differently to information; two individuals receiving identical information may not respond in the same manner.

2. *People are conditioned by their environment and past experiences.* Experiences that interviewees bring with them into an interaction affect their feelings about an interviewer, the situation itself, and any information conveyed.

3. *People behave both verbally and nonverbally on the basis of their needs.* Specific needs that clients bring into an interaction will influence their behavior. What needs do interviewees and counselees have that need to be considered or addressed in a particular interview (to defend, to confirm, to be reassured, to be comforted, or other)?

4. *Needs may be conscious or unconscious.* Are interviewees aware of their needs? Are there unconscious needs that may need to be met?

5. *Needs have both logical and emotional elements.* Many times, an individual's first reactions and overriding feelings about someone or something occur at an emotional level. Logical or rational thinking may occur later. Clinicians who focus primarily or exclusively on rational levels are often unsuccessful, at least initially, when their clients are dealing on more emotional levels.

6. *A person's needs can distort their perceptions and recollections.* An individual's needs may influence or distort what interviewers convey or suggest. This is a primary reason why an expression, such as "but that's not what I said to them," occurs.

7. *People need the recognition, acceptance, and approval of others.* This is important for clinicians to remember—successful interviewers and counselors recognize and affirm others.

8. *People have a need to organize and structure the world.* Donaghy suggests that this is helpful in interviews; it is one reason people are willing to participate in the interviewing and counseling process. Clinicians benefit from people's needs for structure by their participation in these interactions, as well as their assistance in implementing different suggestions. However, interviewees' needs to structure are unproductive if the ways in which they "organize" the world are by stereotyping kinds of attitudes (racially, culturally, genderwise), or other such ramifications; or in attitudes such as therapy is a waste of time, physicians are only out to make money, and so forth.

9. *People have a need to influence the world.* This is a powerful principle—people need to be heard and feel they are influencing an interaction. It is also important in that interviewees who are brought into the clinical treatment process are helping shape their world.

10. *Constructive and lasting changes usually come from satisfying, successful experiences.* One of our critical tasks is to help bring comfort and satisfaction to often troubling situations.

Donaghy (1990) correctly notes that these basic principles only "scratch the surface" of human nature, but the various factors hold important implications for clinicians' interviewing and counseling activities. The discussion of motivation in Chapter 2 also is applicable here with regard to human nature and working effectively with people.

Specific Suggestions for Conveying Information

The following suggestions apply to all interviews in which information is conveyed. This includes discussions following assessment sessions as well as with intervention efforts.

If more than three to five important points need to be made, consider alternative methods for conveying the information. In most cases, another session should be provided on a different occasion when there are many points to be made or there is a series of complex or difficult areas to discuss. Providing a list of the important areas discussed, including a brief comment about each, is also useful. Sending a follow-up letter is also helpful (Martin, 1994). In some settings, an audiocassette recording can also be sent home with participants.

Try to "sandwich" positive and negative points. A "which would you like first, the good news or the bad news?" type of approach is generally inappropriate when conveying information. Conveying all the "good news" first means all the negative information is provided at the end, and that may be what the client retains. On the other hand, if only "bad news" is conveyed first, the interviewee may not hear more positive aspects that are shared later on.

More important, receiving all the positive or the negative aspects at one time hinders developing a true picture of the communicative disorder. Sandwiching the information, on the other hand, allows clients to understand how various findings and factors relate to each other. For example, perhaps we share that a client does have a speech problem because there are too many atypical speech sound errors (an example of bad news). Then we continue by affirming that the child's hearing appears normal and does not account for the problem (an example of good news). By integrating this and additional information, clients begin to get a picture of where the problem lies, what factors are or are not contributing to it, and so forth.

Keep language use simple and appropriate. Professional terminology is complex and not readily understandable for persons without advanced levels of education in the field. The extensiveness of this terminology is illustrated by simply viewing Nicolosi, Harryman, and Kresheck's (1989) *Terminology of Communicative Disorders*—a dictionary that contains over 230 pages of definitions for terms used within the field. Of course, this source does not include all the various possible medical, psychological, and educational terminology that is sometimes used by members of our fields.

Clinicians often use technical terminology on a day-to-day basis and are sometimes unaware when or even how often they use it. Most clients become confused by such professional language. Remember too that clinicians create confusion when they use acronyms, idiosyncratic terms, or terms that are used differently by different specialists (e.g., developmental apraxia and dyspraxia, central auditory processing, or even terms such as mild, moderate, and severe). To minimize confusion, an absolute minimum of technical terminology should be used. When such terms are necessary, or are used inadvertently, they should be defined in everyday language immediately.

"Johnny's *articulation,* his speech sounds . . ."

"Her *diadochokinetic rates,* how quickly she makes rapid speech movements . . ."

"The *rugae,* those prominent ridges right behind his upper teeth . . ."

Be aware that language is not a static entity. Rather, word meanings depend on their context, current usage and, very important, how a listener defines them.

Avoid relying on test names and protocols.   In a majority of cases, people are concerned more with the evaluation or treatment results than with any specific instruments that were used. For example, parents are concerned that a clinician sampled how their child is making speech sounds—it is meaningless that the clinician used the *Arizona, Goldman-Fristoe, Photo Articulation Test, Templin-Darley,* or some other tool for this purpose. The use of test names can also be highly noncommunicative. Saying, "I gave Johnny the *Goldman-Fristoe Test of Articulation* and found three sound errors" is simply less communicative than saying, "I evaluated Johnny's speech sounds and found three sounds that he can't make." The same principle applies for specific procedures and tests used to assess fluency, hearing, language, and voice.

There are some clinicians who feel, perhaps naively, that sharing test protocols (scoring sheets) with clients somehow enhances understanding—but this usually does just the opposite by confusing them. What these individuals fail to realize is that such materials do not mean anything to untrained persons. For example, remember your own confusion and uncertainty the first time you viewed an audiogram, a tympanogram, or the scoring sheets from many language tests.

Luterman (1991) feels that it takes parents of children who are deaf or hearing impaired about a year to really understand an audiogram. Similarly, Martin (1994) suggests that most graphs tend to confuse patients. Throwing out fancy titles or showing test materials or scoresheets is certainly no substitute for appropriate, communicative explanations of your findings. This does not mean that test forms are never to be shared—just do not assume that what is interpretable to a clinician is necessarily understandable to someone else.

Continuously watch for signs of misunderstanding or resistance.   Throughout a session, clinicians need to carefully observe interviewees for verbal and nonverbal signs that they do not understand or are resisting the information being shared. Often, an interviewee's facial expressions or body posture signals that some information is confusing or is not being fully accepted. Such signals are only caught by attending to such factors.

Accept emotional responses professionally, supportively, and matter-of-factly. Being told that there is a problem is an emotional moment for people. Suppose you were told your last five checks had bounced, that your car needed $2,000 worth of repairs, that the one class you needed to graduate had been cancelled, or that the pay raise you were hoping for was denied. All of these are problems that could cause any of us a good deal of emotion at the moment.

Now imagine the emotion involved in being told that a loved one's stroke has caused severe problems understanding others, that a child cannot hear, that a hearing aid will not help, or that long-term therapy is needed. These types of situations are typically accompanied by considerable emotion.

Conversely, consider the opposite range of feelings, those of absolute delight, exhilaration, or relief. People cry at joyous occasions and in pleasant situations—at births, graduations, and weddings; when they win the lottery; when watching a touching story on television or at the movies; among others. Now consider potential reactions if told that there was no problem with a loved one's speech, that a hearing aid would help, or that certain problems could be overcome with assistance. Good news can trigger an emotional release from many people.

Tears and other signs of emotion, whether they are the result of good news or bad news, should be handled matter-of-factly, supportively, and certainly without any criticism. Such expressions of emotionality do not suggest weakness. Clinicians need to have facial tissues available to offer to clients who are affected emotionally. It is also helpful to let the other person know that it is OK to demonstrate such emotion. In most cases, the emotional release is therapeutic.

Other Factors for Effective Communication

There are several other principles interviewers should keep in mind. The following suggestions, which are based on Emerick (1969) and Haynes et al. (1992), are useful when imparting information.

Be alert for emotional static or confusion that inhibits the ability to understand. When either clinicians or those who are interviewed or counseled are feeling anxious or emotionally preoccupied, optimal understanding and communication does not occur. Clinicians should be sensitive to such problems within themselves and with their clients.

Refrain from lecturing or being didactic. Lectures are typically not appreciated in interviewing, counseling, or general conversational situations. Information is obtained from or conveyed to others best when the other party is treated as a "conversational equal." Even better, consider clients and families as partners in the process (Campbell, 1993; Schuyler & Rushmer, 1987; Thornton, 1994).

Not lecturing or being didactic does not, however, imply shirking the responsibility of providing direction and structure to interviewing and counseling situations. A number of clients, including some from linguistically and culturally diverse backgrounds, enter into sessions with the expectation that the authority figure will "control" the situation. Clinicians will need to provide direction, provide specific counsel, and make appropriate recommendations. However, this can be done in conversational and partnership ways that do not involve a one-sided monologue or lecturing the other person.

Use simple language and repeat important words and points. If a client fails to understand assessment findings, treatment results, or recommendations made, it may be immaterial whether any findings are accurate or explanations correct. Using understandable language and employing planned repetitions with varied wordings each time helps ensure successful communication.

Try to provide some constructive action for the party being interviewed. It can be very upsetting for some clients to be told that there is a problem without being given something to do to help resolve the difficulty. This is particularly important if clients cannot be seen for service rather quickly; for example, if a client is placed on a waiting list. It is like telling a student he or she is not doing well in a class. Out of a desire to improve the situation, the student's first question often is, "What can I do to improve my grade?" The client, like the student, wants to do something to improve the situation. Many times, there are some activities or actions that can be suggested.

Present negative information pleasantly but candidly. Martin (1994) comments that "the skill with which 'bad news' is initially delivered may have a profound effect on acceptance of the disorder and all the efforts toward rehabilitation that become necessary" (p. 39). It can be difficult to present bad news, but it is inappropriate to provide false assurances or to fail to convey findings and impressions accurately and honestly. Say what needs to be said kindly but candidly. The presentation of negative information sometimes needs to be preceded with more positive aspects of the situation, particularly with some individuals from cultures that place value on degrees of indirectness (e.g., Filipino or native American).

Some cultures, such as the European American culture, are relatively direct and "to the point." Other cultures are less direct. However, degrees of directness generally refer to how information is conveyed, and information that precedes or prefaces certain presentations. Across cultures, clinicians still need to convey what has to be said—the differences are in how and in what order clinicians do this.

Realize that the "bearer of bad news" may be subjected to an interviewee's anger or other negative reactions. Anyone can be blamed for something—a physician may be blamed for identifying a serious disorder, an innocent store clerk verbally assaulted for the high costs of products, or a meal server criticized for "cooking" a bad meal. Clinicians are often the most available person for clients or their caregivers involved with a communicative disorder to "dump on." Secure clinicians are prepared to serve as an emotional lightning rod for clients, if needed. Clinicians are aware that many ventilations of anger and other feelings, although they may be expressed at the professional, are not really aimed at or caused by them (Hutchinson, 1979).

Whenever possible and appropriate, provide encouragement to clients and family members. Interviews tend to result in more positive action when strengths and possibilities are emphasized rather than weaknesses and limitations. Sometimes, a client's mere acknowledgment that there may be a problem is an important first step in the overall picture.

Don't be surprised if some suggestions are not acted on immediately. Not everyone will heed advice or suggestions made (Mowrer, 1988; Shipley & Wood, 1996). If well-intended, sound advice were always taken, there would be far fewer unwanted pregnancies, people would not smoke, alcohol and drugs would not be abused, and so forth. The same principle applies to communicative disorders. Not every patient will follow exactly what the professional suggests.

From time to time, there are a few clients who seek confirmation of their own feelings and conclusions—irrespective of what a clinician says or what others in the field have said. Some of these persons will fail to accept clinicians' findings and recommendations, and they will continue to seek confirmation of their beliefs elsewhere.

Concluding Comments

An information-giving interview, like the information-getting interview, can be seen as proceeding through three distinct phases—an opening, the body, and a closing. By approaching the interview systematically in terms of these three phases and working at smooth transitions between the segments, clinicians minimize confusion and reduce awkward moments of undirected conversation.

A clinician's preparation for an information-giving interview is important. The interviewer should carefully choose the major points to be shared with an eye toward avoiding information overload. Three to five points is often a good general rule. Clinicians should also plan the presentation of specific observations and general conclusions in relation to an interviewee's emotional state, such as whether they are highly anxious about information they anticipate will be presented.

Just as important for the success of providing information is the skill with which clinicians communicate their information and suggestions to clients—balancing good and bad news, choosing the language to use carefully, staying alert for signs of confusion or misunderstanding, and dealing professionally with emotional responses. The closing phase of the interview provides a final opportunity for a clinician to summarize and clarify points for the client's understanding.

C h a p t e r 7

Areas of Counseling

Counseling is an important aspect of clinical work. In their professional practices, clinicians engage frequently in counseling activities—whether they call it interviewing, helping, or counseling. They discuss communicative disorders, their effects, and their treatment with clients, families and other caregivers. Clinicians provide ideas and methods for promoting communicative growth and methods for coping with different problems. They help clients and families release or identify feelings related to communicative difficulties, help people adjust to or cope better with their difficulties, and then face new challenges and develop new skills.

Stated differently, one role of counseling activities is to help clients adjust to current situations, to help them cope with a communicative disorder and its ramifications in life. Another function is to help patients and caregivers release "pent up" frustrations and deal with their lives in more productive manners. A third basic function is to facilitate learning; in effect, teaching clients or caregivers more about a particular disorder or its treatment. A fourth function is to help alter or modify people's feelings, attitudes, or behaviors that are helping maintain a communicative disorder, or are counterproductive to improving the problem.

In other words, clinicians seek to bring about for clients greater understanding of themselves, their feelings, their environments, their communicative disorders and the disorders' effects, and changes that are necessary to improve their situations. Clinicians, therefore, need to develop the skills necessary to enable such understanding and promote changes that are considered appropriate.

Counseling Defined

Counseling in audiology and speech-language pathology has been defined as advising, directing, and exchanging opinions and ideas (Scheuerle, 1992). It has also been considered within the context of informing, persuading, or listening to and valuing others (Luterman, 1991). Counseling is defined here quite simply as a helping relationship that involves one party who needs help, another party who provides help, and a setting that allows a helping process to occur (Cormier & Hackney, 1987). Counseling involves a number of different functions. It is certainly more than some "standard" set of procedures; counseling is a process that includes a series of caring and purposeful actions to achieve preselected and specific objectives and goals (Purkey & Schmidt, 1987).

Characteristics of Good Counselors

An important characteristic of counselors in our field is willingness to expand personal boundaries, to learn and experience more so that patients and families will benefit. A variety of other skills and attitudes characterize an effective counselor. The characteristics reviewed in Chapter 2—spontaneity, flexibility, concentration, openness, honesty, emotional stability, trustworthiness, self-awareness, belief in the client's ability to change, commitment to helping people change, wisdom, communication skills, professional competence—are important for effective counseling.

Years ago, Erickson (1950) wrote that good counselors need to use a variety of methods and approaches, be able to shift from one method to another when appropriate, use the tools that work best for the client, be highly skilled, and remain skilled by continued study and self-improvement. These characteristics remain of paramount importance today. As DeBlassie (1976) comments, a counselor

> Is a unique individual who is creative, has a profound belief in the dignity and worth of the individual, is open-minded, has a tolerance for ambiguity, is experienced in counseling with others, is spontaneous and flexible, is knowledgeable about self and others, has a thorough knowledge of the behavioral sciences, and has a deep commitment toward helping people. (p. 92)

More recently, Biggs and Blocher (1987) comment that

> Nothing is more central to the practice of counseling . . . than trust. Counseling, by its very nature, involves a relationship built on mutual confidence, respect, and consideration. . . . To a considerable degree, however, the clinician not only depends on his or her own clinical skills and communication of expertness, attractiveness, and trustworthiness but also draws on the generalized expectations of trustworthiness, expertness, and integrity that the client

brings to the counseling situation from his or her own experiences as a member of the larger society. (p. 65)

Counseling in Educational and Clinical Settings

The Need for Counseling

The need for effective counseling as a part of the assessment or treatment with communicative disorders is noted in a number of audiology and speech-language pathology textbooks. Unfortunately, however, the sections dealing with counseling are often limited, sometimes simply to general recommendations to provide counseling if it is needed. There are relatively few discussions of how to counsel, or even the specific areas that should be addressed. The need for counseling is also suggested in a variety of journal articles. Again, however, it is generally assumed that readers will already know what or how to counsel.

Despite widespread agreement about the need for interviewing and counseling abilities, these skills are often neglected within professional preparation programs and clinical and research literature (Clark, 1994a; Colton & Casper, 1990; Gregory, 1995; Hegde, 1993; Hutchinson, 1979; Culpepper, Mendel, & McCarthy, 1994; Johnson, 1994; McFarlane, Fujiki, & Brinton, 1984, and others). Stone and Olswang (1989) comment that

> *Counseling and family involvement in treatment of communication disorders are not new activities per se, though current applications are expanded and innovative. . . . Despite counseling's historical and continuing place in communicative disorders, many professionals remain uncomfortable with counseling responsibilities. Uncertainty persists as to where counseling fits into communication disorders works. . . . Such uncertainty may be because few speech-language pathologists and audiologists receive adequate educational preparation in counseling, since counseling courses are significantly underrepresented in standard speech and hearing curricula. . . . Thus, although most speech-language pathologists and audiologists agree on the importance of counseling, they may feel they lack the necessary tools to incorporate counseling into their work.* (p. 27)

Webster and Ward (1993) outline the following four major functions of communicative disorders specialists who work with parents:

1. Obtaining information
2. Giving information
3. Understanding and clarifying ideas, attitudes, emotions, and behaviors
4. Offering alternatives for personal behavior, or the behavior of others, and assisting in making these changes. (Adapted from pp. 4-5.)

These functions apply, not just to parents, but to clients irrespective of age. Obtaining and providing information are discussed in Chapters 5 and 6. The understanding and clarification of ideas, attitudes, emotions, and behaviors, as well as assisting people in making changes, is addressed primarily in this chapter.

Counseling activities can focus on the past by addressing what has occurred, on the present by addressing what is currently happening, or on the future by determining and promoting what needs to be done. Years ago, Irwin (1969) described some of the counseling roles clinicians assume when serving parents of children with speech-language disorders. She felt that clinicians could help parents within twelve areas, including:

1. Facing facts about themselves and their children.
2. Gaining understanding of mental health in relation to speech and hearing problems.
3. Observing children's verbal behavior sympathetically and with understanding.
4. Learning how to record observations of children's behavior.
5. Learning how to react to the behavior of children with objectivity and understanding.
6. Learning the best scientific information on speech, hearing, and behavior problems through selected readings and discussions.
7. Learning how to apply some of the basic principles of general semantics in parent-child relationships.
8. Learning how to use the scientific method of solving problems.
9. Learning specific speech and hearing techniques that may be used at home.
10. Gaining an understanding of verbal behavior and speech stimuli which affect children's speech and language.
11. Minimizing or reducing feelings of isolation and difference.
12. Releasing anxiety. (Adapted from Irwin, 1969, p. 16.)

Clearly these are important functions with many clients, both young and old, and with many families and other caregivers. It should be noted that, within Irwin's (1969) listing of counseling areas, both *informational* and *affective* functions are found. Sometimes counseling is a matter of educating; other times counseling is directed more toward helping interviewees ventilate their feelings and reducing "blocks" that aggravate a patient's or family's situation.

Guidance, Counseling, and Psychotherapy

Besides lacking formal preparation for counseling, many clinicians experience uncertainty concerning the boundaries of counseling. How, for example, is counseling different than providing guidance or than psychotherapy? Each of these three activities is different, yet they sometimes overlap, causing role confusion for clinicians.

Guidance, counseling, and psychotherapy should be viewed as activities on a continuum rather than as well-defined, distinct practices (Mowrer, 1988; Rollin, 1987). Mowrer (1988) notes that each of these functions is really a process. The process of guidance generally involves providing information to people; counseling involves helping people solve problems by doing more than simply providing information; psychotherapy involves helping individuals make more profound personal adjustments. The area of counseling helps an otherwise normal person make certain adjustments. *Psychotherapy* is more concerned with the treatment of psychological abnormality, treatment that encourages considerable individual adjustment, sometimes even basic personality changes. Using a medical model, Rollin (1987) feels that individuals requiring psychotherapy are "sick" and need help to alter psychopathological feelings and behavior. Thus, psychotherapy generally falls within the province of psychiatry, clinical psychology, or other mental health professions.

Counseling has to do with personal adjustment rather than with major personality changes. Counseling helps people examine their methods or styles of interacting with others, analyze their positive and counterproductive behaviors, evaluate and face their values and beliefs, increase their personal awareness and self-knowledge, and achieve self-development (DeBlassie, 1976). As Luterman (1991) comments:

> *The aim of counseling is to help the client [or family] become more congruent in order to contend successfully with the problem at hand. Counseling as practiced by speech pathologists and audiologists should be problem centered with otherwise normal individuals who are emotionally upset by the problem at hand. This is opposed to psychotherapy, the province of specially trained professionals who are dealing with people who have chronic life adjustment problems. Many of the skills needed by both counselors and psychotherapists overlap considerably. It is the nature of the client and the nature of the problem that differ.* (p. 5)

Guidance is a method of influencing another person's thoughts or behaviors that is typically less formal than counseling or psychotherapy. Guidance may or may not be provided by someone with advanced or specific training. Generally, guidance involves an educational process in which information is dispensed (Mowrer, 1988). Advice may be given, suggestions may be offered, informational materials may be distributed, and so forth.

Speech-language pathologists and audiologists are ideally suited to provide guidance and many types of counseling because of their intensive training in rehabilitative procedures, and because they work directly and intensively with individuals who have disabilities (Mowrer, 1988). In her classic article about counseling parents, Webster (1966) addresses an important question faced by professionals treating communicative disorders:

The question sometimes arises, "Can't the speech pathologist or audiologist do damage to parents by attempting to counsel with them?" The answer depends in part on how one defines counseling. If counseling means the imposition of prescriptions without care for the person for whom they are prescribed, one may indeed do damage. The nonaccepting, noncompassionate clinician runs the risk of hurting parents; so does the one who focuses concern on the child to the exclusion of concern for the parents. The speech pathologist or audiologist who leaves to others the interpretation of the information his [or her] field has to offer may do parents great harm. The same can be said for the clinician with limited knowledge who gives faulty information. (p. 339)

Professionals treating communicative disorders need counseling skills in order to serve the best interests of their clients. Counseling is being used more and more in the treatment of communicative disorders and in new and different ways, so clinicians must remain flexible and willing to work with various counseling theories, approaches, and procedures (Stone & Olswang, 1989). However, speech and hearing professionals also need to be aware of their limitations as counselors (Hutchinson, 1979). It is critical that clinicians have the judgment to know when their training and experience will not suffice, and when they should make referrals to professionals with more specialized counseling or psychotherapeutic training. This leads to considering the concept of boundaries.

Boundaries of Counseling

ASHA's (1990) *Scope of Practice* specifically mentions counseling as an appropriate function of speech-language pathologists and audiologists. Stone and Olswang (1989) note that, while there has long been a need for professionals in our field to involve themselves in counseling activities, there are also somewhat pervasive "discomfort levels" about counseling—What it is? Who should do it? What it should entail or encompass? When should it be done? Stone and Olswang appropriately note that much of this discomfort originates from two sources: our professions' general lack of preprofessional exposure to counseling, and to the question of boundaries. What are, for example, the roles and responsibilities of professionals in communicative disorders, and what are the roles and responsibilities of other professionals (psychologists, mental health counselors, social workers, etc.)? It is important to understand our roles as well as those roles that are best served by others. Some of the information in the following paragraphs is based on Stone and Olswang's (1989) contribution.

Knowing one's boundaries does not occur in a single lesson, rather, they change and (hopefully) expand across time. Boundaries are related to the individual clinician and that person's skills and abilities, the setting in which the person works, and the clients being served and their needs. For example, clinicians working in settings or geographic locations where mental health specialists are not readily available will involve themselves in activities that other individuals who have greater access to psychologists, counselors, or other mental health professionals will not. Some of the basic goals of most counseling include: (1) establishing an environment within which change can occur; (2) providing information about communicative disorders and their remediation; (3) providing release and support for those who need it; and (4) assisting in the improvement or resolution of patients' or families' problems, particularly as they pertain to a communicative disorder.

These are all activities that fall within the domain or province of professionals in communicative disorders, particularly as problems relate to a communicative problem or its effects. However, counseling intended to make major personality adjustments or change someone's basic response patterns to events in life typically are best handled by an appropriately trained mental health professional. Again using a medical model, psychotherapy deals with a "sick" individual (Luterman, 1991; Rollin, 1987). The counseling we do helps people adapt to, live with, and work toward improving a communicative problem and its ramifications.

There are "internally" and "externally" defined boundaries that define roles in counseling. Internally defined boundaries relate to how individuals perceive their own abilities and skills. "I can help with that" or "I need to help my client address _____," versus "I can't talk with them about _____ " or "That's not my job" are examples of internally defined boundaries. Good clinicians work to expand their internally defined boundaries and, thus, serve their patients better.

Externally defined boundaries refer to some limitation placed on a clinician by external forces. Not trying to assist a patient overcome a phobia of heights or of snakes or spiders is an externally defined boundary—such help customarily and appropriately falls within the province of a mental health professional. A restrictive job description or the expectations of colleagues in a work setting are also examples of externally defined boundaries.

Either internally or externally defined boundaries can influence what the counselor does with patients. In general, our role is to expand boundaries—whether internal of external—so that we can provide the services needed by our patients and families. Boundaries change, particularly as clinicians acquire greater skills and abilities and experience, and as other people see how effective professionals in communicative disorders can be with different situations or problems.

Internally or externally defined boundaries can influence the content of counseling efforts. Attitudes, behaviors, information, and problems associated with communicative disorders are clearly within our province. Who else, for example, knows more about these areas than audiologists and speech-language pathologists? Areas that are beyond speech and hearing clinician's boundaries include subjects such as unrelated medical problems, chronic unhappiness and depression, marital instability, and domestic violence (Stone & Olswang, 1989). These authors note that some areas—interpersonal relations between persons with a communicative disorder and significant others, a client's deep grieving about a communicative disorder, difficulties adjusting to a communicative disorder, and helping with behavior management with communicatively disordered children—often "test the boundaries" within which we work. However, other authorities (e.g., Leith, 1993) see speech-language pathologists in particular as being among the best persons available to assist with these types of problems. Certainly when such problems are related to a communicative disorder, the speech and hearing specialist can be extremely helpful.

Approaches to Counseling

All approaches to counseling have the person-to-person nature of the work in common. Counseling, as we have defined it, is a helping relationship in which one participant assumes the responsibility of helping the other. It is further assumed that both participants see the welfare of the one being helped as the central concern of the relationship, and that the participants will work together toward solutions to problems that influence that welfare. In the case of a clinician counseling a young patient's parents, of course, it is the welfare of a third party—the child—that is the central concern.

The speech and hearing fields do not have unique or distinctively different approaches to counseling than other fields. Indeed, our professionals have relied on different approaches initially developed for use in psychology and other counseling professions. It is beyond the scope of this book to describe all the different approaches that have been developed over the years, and it is not necessary. For readers who are interested in the different approaches, Meier and Davis' (1993) *The Elements of Counseling* contains a brief description of the major counseling types in a readable, introductory manner. Other resources containing more information include Brammer (1993); Brammer, Abrego, and Shostrom (1993); Engelkes and Vandergoot (1982); Mowrer (1988); Okun (1992); Rollin (1987); Woody, Hansen, and Rossberg (1989); or others. The approaches most frequently useful in speech and hearing are described in the sections that follow. But first, let's consider the notions of direct and indirect approaches to helping.

Directive and Nondirective Approaches

An important way in which counseling approaches vary is in the degree of direction that counselors provide to clients. In directive (or active) approaches, it is the clinician who takes major responsibility for assessing the problems encountered and for focusing any intervention or treatment (Stewart & Cash, 1994). These counselors play an active role in directing the discussions and activities of intervention. In nondirective approaches, on the other hand, the client plays a greater role in determining the problems at hand and their possible solutions. Nondirective methodologies tend to stress the creation of an atmosphere in which clients engage in explorations of their feelings, self-explorations that ultimately lead them to their own healthful conclusions about themselves, others, and the problems at hand.

Nondirective approaches are often associated with the client-centered therapy advocated by Carl Rogers (1951, 1986). In client-centered counseling the client is encouraged to take most of the responsibility for providing direction to the interactions. This approach is potentially useful for professionals who need to help clients release pent-up emotions, clarify specific feelings, understand certain reactions, and learn to accept certain problems. However, this form of counseling, when it is used, is generally more appropriate in psychotherapy than in the treatment of most communicative disorders.

Directive approaches are useful when clinicians are reasonably sure of a problem and appropriate alternatives for its treatment. Such is the case in most clinical activities in communicative disorders because speech-language pathologists or audiologists typically know what the disorder is and what course of action is needed. In these cases, a form of directive counseling allows clinicians to share information and to work more directly toward modifying certain feelings, attitudes, and behavior that are connected to the disorder.

Client-Centered Approaches

It has already been noted that client-centered approaches are typically associated with Carl Rogers's work in psychotherapy. These approaches are generally indirect, placing primary responsibility for providing direction, and even some structure to interactions, on clients. There are clinical situations in communicative disorders for which it is helpful to yield responsibility for direction to clients who need to work out personal feelings and reactions. However, the use of this approach does require specific training, and as Mowrer (1977) commented some years ago, client-centered counseling is considered valuable by some but it certainly takes a backseat to newer approaches. Thus, client-centered or more indirect approaches are not often seen in speech-language pathology and audiology. They take special skills, the availability of considerable time, and usually a series of relatively frequent contacts with patients. There are also more effective approaches for most clients, particularly the more direct behavioral and cognitively based approaches.

Behavioral Counseling

Behavioral counseling grew out of the work of B. F. Skinner and those who followed him in operant learning and conditioning. The movement toward behavioral counseling is a significant departure from previous counseling approaches, which were for the most part phenomenological (i.e., subjective, intentional, motive-oriented). A behavioral approach to counseling is generally distinguished by its focus on specifically identifiable attitudes or behavior of clients, rather than on presumed "deep" underlying causes of those attitudes or behavior.

The focus is on what can be observed and measured objectively—behavior understood as the outward manifestation of feelings and attitudes—rather than on the subjectively determined, speculative, or unknown origins of a problem. Under this type of approach to counseling, behavior is often defined as including only objectively or publicly observable responses. That behavior is understood as being a response means that it can be learned through the use of operant conditioning methods—through, that is, positive reinforcement, negative reinforcement, and/or punishment of responses elicited. This is an important premise of the behavioral approach to counseling.

A behavioral approach to counseling is very attractive to professionals treating communicative disorders because it allows them to focus on areas that affect a client's communicative abilities. In other words, clinicians can focus primarily on feelings, attitudes, or behaviors that pertain directly to communicative difficulties, thus limiting themselves to areas for which they have had proper training and experience. Furthermore, clinicians are already well trained in and knowledgeable about the various techniques that effectively promote change. Using a behavioral model, they implement consistent procedures that utilize appropriate shaping techniques and procedures to alter clients' behavior or to influence clients' feelings and attitudes.

A behavioral approach also is appealing to clinicians because the effects of counseling can be measured on an ongoing basis. By evaluating behaviors before and after sessions, or following a series of sessions, clinicians monitor the effectiveness of their counseling efforts. Finally, behavioral approaches are attractive because they are very effective!

Krumboltz and Thoresen (1969), pioneers in behavioral counseling, describe the four essential features of a behavioral orientation: (1) selecting a goal, (2) tailoring specific procedures and techniques to meet the client's needs, (3) experimenting with various techniques while simultaneously assessing their effectiveness, and (4) monitoring feedback from the counseling session constantly. These features are familiar to clinicians in communicative disorders because they are fundamental to most clinical intervention activities. Behavioral approaches are well-grounded and useful because of the following:

- The basic principles, being empirically derived, are based on observation and experience.
- The effectiveness of behavioral techniques for altering behavior makes them ideal in clinical settings where the effects of specific behaviors can be pinpointed.
- Behavioral techniques produce observable data to support the effectiveness of intervention. (Adapted from Brown & Brown, 1975; and Hegde, 1993.)

A behavioral approach allows clinicians to select goals and objectives to be achieved through the counseling efforts. Whenever possible, counselors and counselees should agree on goals that are attainable and measurable. The orientation does not call for the exclusive use of a single procedure or specific set of procedures. Rather, counselors employ a variety of possible techniques to alter or influence behavior and attitudes. Many appropriate reinforcement or punishment procedures can be employed. Clinicians can also use various teaching methods such as direct instruction, modeling, feedback, and providing specific suggestions. Behaviorally based counseling allows clinicians to evaluate different techniques employed, the effects of which can be determined through the results of counseling efforts on an ongoing basis—after one session or after a series of sessions, after a week or a month or three months, and so forth (Krumboltz & Thoresen, 1969).

Cognitive Approaches

Another effective counseling model is the cognitive approach, which is not always separate from a behavioral approach. A cognitively based form of counseling is often used as a general term, encompassing what have been called constructivism, rational-emotive therapy, reality therapy, and cognitive/behavioral therapies (Okun, 1992). Meier and Davis (1993) discuss the cognitive approaches under a category that includes cognitive, cognitive/behavioral, and social learning counseling. The essence of most cognitive approaches, at least for the purposes here, is that a person's thoughts—particularly those that are harmful, inappropriate, or counterproductive—cause or at least contribute to harmful; painful; or counterproductive feelings, attitudes, or behavior. Leith (1993) provides the following useful example about:

> ... a stutterer who feels that when he stutters, everyone stops what they are doing and looks at him. He will not order food in a restaurant because everyone will hear him, look at him, watch him as he completes his order, and discuss him with others at their table. He feels that he becomes the center of attention when he stutters. If the waitress stands across from him to take his order, he is even more intimidated since, if he speaks up, all of the people in the restaurant will turn and look at him. ... (p. 208)

With a patient like this, there are two problems—the stuttering behaviors themselves and the rather intense, self-conscious feelings about being dysfluent. It is possible that, even if this client's dysfluencies were reduced or eliminated, at least some of the intense feelings about "always being watched" would remain. Thus, a cognitive approach is used to modify or eliminate some of these harmful and counterproductive feelings. This is done through counseling by (1) identifying and focusing on the precise problem area, (2) identifying the distorted thoughts (cognitions), (3) confronting the problem area with new thought (cognitive orientations), and (4) changing the thought (cognitive set) by objectively evaluating the new thoughts.

Using Leith's (1993) example, the clinician would proceed through these steps by:

1. *Identifying the problem area*—how the client perceives the stuttering and how "everyone in the world is watching and talking about it" when it happens.

2. *Identifying the distortions involved*—everyone really is watching and that, subsequently, this will be the source of everyone's conversation, ridicule, feelings of pity, or whatever.

3. *Confronting the problem area with new thoughts*—for example, others in the restaurant are really preoccupied with their own concerns, half the restaurant could not hear the conversation anyway, and so on. In effect, more logical and real thoughts are used in place of more emotionally based, distorted thoughts.

4. *Changing the old belief system (cognitive set)* to new, more realistic and appropriate thoughts through evaluation. Perhaps the client is instructed to order at a restaurant and, when stuttering does occur, observe that indeed the whole world has not stopped to observe. In fact, most of them were not even listening.

Cognitive approaches are used frequently in various mental health counseling activities; they are also useful with speech and hearing. Basic thoughts are reshaped into more constructive feelings and attitudes. For example, parents who "would be of no help whatsoever" are approached with new attitudes and feelings—yes, they can help and will be of immense assistance. Just a few other examples include the following:

"No the hearing aid is not the first thing everyone notices."

"Yes, you can play on the playground without shouting."

"Many children have speech problems; you're not the only one in the world."

"A slower, more controlled, fluent speech rate sounds normal and good—not like some robot."

"We're looking for intelligible speech rather than *perfect* speech."

"Every journey begins with the first step," "Rome wasn't built in a day," and so forth.

Again, cognitive approaches are helpful for a variety of situations and problems. These approaches are often used in combination with certain support groups or readings. For example, books, such as John-Roger and McWilliams' (1992) *The Portable Life 101,* are particularly useful with some patients, particularly those with more negative cognitive sets (e.g., the glass is always half-empty rather than half-full).

Cognitive/Behavioral Approaches

Cognitive/behavioral models are simply combinations of the behavioral and cognitive approaches. Specific feelings and attitudes are addressed by using elements of both approaches. This is frequently the most powerful and effective combination available. Consider the following example: Ann Landers, the syndicated advice columnist, printed a list of the "Seven Steps to Stagnation" several years ago. This list, by an unknown author, includes:

1. We've never done it that way.
2. We're not ready for that yet.
3. We're doing all right without it.
4. We tried it once, and it didn't work out.
5. It costs too much.
6. That's not our responsibility.
7. It won't work.

These factors, which most readers will identify having heard before and which many clinicians encounter in one form or another, are areas that may require attention before optimal progress is possible. Such feelings are often modifiable through counseling that includes a combination of the cognitive and behavioral principles described in the previous sections.

The Process of Counseling

One type of counseling is providing information, so the processes and techniques of giving information described in Chapter 6 apply to these types of interactions. Activities that are intended to help patients or caregivers understand or clarify their feelings, attitudes, emotions, or behaviors—or activities offering these individuals methods and alternatives for changing behavior—are typically viewed as being more within the "counseling" realm. The information in the following sections describes the basic stages or processes available for these types of interactions. These basic steps are used irrespective of any particular counseling approach employed (behavioral, cognitive, cognitive/behavioral, or most others).

Depending on the authority consulted, the process of counseling has anywhere from two to more than ten steps (see, for example, Brammer et al., 1993; Cormier & Hackney, 1987; DeBlassie, 1976; Hackney

& Cormier, 1994; Moursund, 1993; Okun, 1992; Schum, 1986). For example, Okun (1992) views counseling as a two-step process. The first stage involves building a relationship so it includes establishing rapport, developing trust, encouraging client self-disclosure, listening, attending, and so forth. The second stage involves strategic planning, implementation, evaluation, termination, and follow-up.

DeBlassie (1976), on the other hand, outlines the following eight steps in the counseling process.

1. Observing the situation.
2. Ordering and assessing observations.
3. Predicting the course of events without intervention.
4. Predicting the course of events with intervention.
5. Formulating tentative hypotheses and alternatives.
6 Providing purposeful intervention.
7. Observing the effects of intervention.
8. Reassessing previous appraisals and reformulating hypotheses. (Adapted from DeBlassie, 1976, p. 87.)

These basic steps provide excellent guidelines for determining the need for counseling, developing and providing appropriate counseling, and evaluating the effects of clinical efforts. It is also worth noting that these eight steps can be applied to any clinical activities, including diagnostic or treatment sessions.

Although various authorities have outlined different numbers of stages in the counseling process, these differences relate more to how specific each step is than to actual differences in the process. For example, Okun (1992), as we have seen, includes activities like planning, implementing, evaluating, terminating, and following up within the second of her two stages, whereas other authorities would consider each of these activities a separate stage in the process.

My preference is to use Cormier and Hackney's (1987) five-stage model for counseling activities (see Figure 7.1). The stages in this model can overlap so that, for example, clinicians may continue to build relationships across any of the stages. The model is also sequential in that it moves progressively from building a relationship to assessment, to goal-setting, to counseling intervention, to eventual termination and follow-up.

The Counseling Session

Preparation

Adequate preparation is as critical for counseling as it is for other types of interviewing, if not more so. Clinicians should begin their preparation by carefully considering the information available and the insights already gained about those involved with counseling efforts. This includes

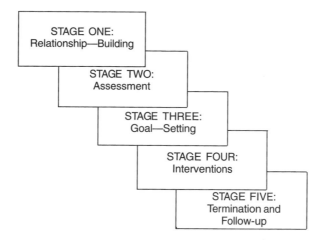

FIGURE 7.1 The Stages of Counseling

Source: From *The Professional Counselor: A Process Guide to Helping* (p. 19) by L. S. Cormier and H. Hackney, 1987, Englewood Cliffs, NJ: Prentice-Hall. Copyright 1987 by Prentice-Hall, Inc. Reprinted by permission.

a client's communicative disorder, any particular reactions or feelings of concern, or other areas that need attention. Through this study clinicians begin to plan how to orient the client; how to establish rapport; how to set the tone for one or more interactions; how to communicate understanding to the other party; what information to provide; and what specific attitudes, feelings, or behaviors to address. To allow for adequate preparation, advance appointments are recommended. As a standard part of preparation, attention should also be paid to the physical environment. The counseling space should appear professional and allow for privacy and comfort.

Beginning a Session

With adequate preparation, the clinician should have a fairly clear idea of what needs to be done during a session, and begins the initial counseling by describing the basic structure of the interaction for the client. The initial structuring information should include a description of the purpose of the meeting—for example, what is the problem to be addressed. It is also helpful to describe what general results a counseling session may be expected to achieve. If a clinician has initiated the session, it is a good idea to begin the meeting with a brief explanation of why the client is being involved. If sessions have been initiated by counselees, it is helpful to let them begin by explaining why they have requested the session (Brown & Brown, 1975; Stewart & Cash, 1994).

"I'm glad we have this chance to talk together. I know you have been very concerned about your husband's speech. You were kind enough to share that you were frustrated with his progress. Perhaps you could share some of these frustrations. Then, I think I may have a couple of suggestions for you. Tell me about some of your concerns."

"I've been concerned about how you are feeling about your stuttering. It seems like you feel the whole world is listening to your every word. There are some things you may be perceiving a little incorrectly. I want to talk about several of these. A little later, I do have two things I'd like you to try. First, let's talk about _____ ."

"I'm glad you scheduled this appointment. It's good to have a chance to talk about _____ . What are some of the things on your mind?"

Such wordings are only examples; they can be modified as appropriate to different situations. When participants are involved in ongoing counseling sessions, clinicians need to begin each new session by reviewing overall expectations and reassessing previous discussions and activities. Such orientations help ensure that both parties are on common ground.

The Content of Counseling

Meier and Davis (1993) point out that psychologists and other mental health counselors typically talk about three systems: affect, cognition, and behavior. *Affect* refers to feelings. The "big four" feelings are anger, sadness, fear, and joy (Meier & Davis, 1993). *Cognitions* refer to thoughts. For example, "I can't do it," "This is too difficult," "She's not getting any better," "It's all my fault that she is stuttering." "If I had only _____ ." *Behaviors* refer to some type of actions. For example, a dysfluency, a harsh glottal attack, changing the subject abruptly, doing or not doing home activities, wearing or not wearing the hearing aid, and so forth.

The topics discussed during a counseling session may be in any one, two, or even all three of these systems. This will depend on the needs of the client, the client's family, or other caregivers. Webster (1968) discusses the importance of counseling with parents of communicatively impaired children and suggests that counseling can benefit such parents in at least three ways. First, it can help them understand their own feelings and emotions that relate to the situation at hand, and this enlarged understanding can lead them to more effective interactions with their child. Second, counseling can provide important information to parents, information that increases their understanding of what needs to be done. Third, counseling can provide parents with tools to help them communicate more effectively with each other and with their child. Counseling can bring these same benefits to spouses, adult children, and others. Any of these three benefits may occur by focusing on specific affect, cognitions, and/or behaviors that need addressing.

Of course, for any given counseling session, clinicians must determine which areas will be most beneficial to counselees. Then, for example, if a clinician's purpose is to provide the client with more information about a communicative disorder, this information will be the major content of the counseling session. If the clinician needs for counselees to change their attitudes or behavior toward someone with a communicative difficulty, modifying these responses will be the primary counseling content.

In Chapter 6, it was suggested that the content of information-giving interviews should be limited to three to five major points. For counselors, there may be one or many major points made, problems discussed, feelings expressed and understood, or behaviors or attitudes targeted for modification. When there are multiple areas that require attention, counselors are advised to limit the topics to a reasonable number within any particular interaction. Introducing too many areas for consideration at a given time can be confusing and may preclude understanding of them. If too many topics are addressed during a session, some or even all of them may be too superficially addressed for any good to occur. Additional topics are sometimes best introduced at different times along a counseling treatment sequence.

Closing the Interview

Interviews in which clinicians are providing information, giving instruction, or in other ways trying to promote some form of change are often closed in a fashion similar to the information-giving interviews as described in Chapter 6. This includes summarizing the major points discussed; soliciting questions; expressing appreciation for clients' help, interest, and/or participation; and reviewing any next steps that will be involved.

Sessions in which a patient or caregiver is doing most of the talking—expressing feelings, releasing and ventilating feelings, and/or receiving a clinicians' support—usually require some advance warning when the time allotted is about to expire. Most counselors recommend preparing clients for the end of a session five to ten minutes before the time is actually over. This is done with statements or questions such as "Our time is about up. Is there something else you wanted to consider?" or "We have about ten more minutes. Are there areas you wanted to talk about further?" Cues help clients begin the process of ending a session, and are certainly preferable to ending with something like "Oh, our time is up. We'll talk further _____." When time does expire, these sessions are also closed in the manner described in the previous paragraph.

Aspects of Counseling

Conditioning Attitudes and Behavior

After clinicians determine which attitudes or behaviors require attention, promoting desired change often involves providing the information that is needed and, as appropriate, providing the rationales that support this information. Clinicians need to communicate to clients an understanding of what needs to be changed, and why.

Clinicians then set about conditioning actual behaviors and attitudes, using appropriate shaping procedures including reinforcement or punishment. In operant terms, changes in a desired direction are reinforced while changes away from a desired direction are not reinforced and/or are punished. Reinforcement and punishment techniques affect the frequency of activities in that properly implemented reinforcers increase target attitudes or behavior, whereas appropriately administered punishers decrease the frequency of these feelings or behaviors. A number of specific verbal and nonverbal methods useful for conditioning behavior are addressed in Chapter 4.

Explaining Behavioral Principles

Many counselors teach basic behavioral concepts to counselees, particularly when parents or other caregivers are involved in helping reinforce or extinguish behaviors. In these cases, it is important for the people involved to understand the elements of basic conditioning and shaping. Years ago, Brown and Brown (1975) described the teaching of operant conditioning to parents and suggested that:

> *Parents quickly grasp these principles if a common sense approach is used. Obviously, positive reinforcement might be explained as an event that increases the probability of a behavior occurring again in the future. However, parents readily understand that money and food act as rewards and are thus influential in the motivation of behavior. They also understand that individuals respond to pats on the back, smiles, and caresses when the idea is put to them simply. We usually ask parents what they respond to or what makes them feel like doing something again. When parents begin to talk about the things that reinforce them, they begin to understand the concept more clearly. Once positive reinforcement is understood, the idea of extinction can also be explained. This explanation is often prefaced by a question such as "What would happen if someone stopped paying you to go to work?" It is also important to illustrate to parents that devices often seen as punishment (e.g., threatening the child) may in fact be rewarding and reinforce behavior, since the child thus receives attention for his or her behavior. The concept of negative reinforcement can be introduced by asking parents to relate their reaction whenever they yell at a noisy child and the noise ceases.* (p. 99)

As this example illustrates, descriptions of basic behavioral techniques should be tailored to the situation of the counselee and worded in ways that assure understanding.

Providing Advice

Many counseling activities involve sharing information within preselected areas. Clinicians should remember that advice must be based on sound and adequate information. They should not provide advice or guidance if there is uncertainty about the information, or if the areas discussed are beyond the bounds of their knowledge and professional training.

Having Reasonable Expectations

Years ago, Cozad (1974) described the notion of being reasonable regarding expectations for some children with hearing impairments. The same principle applies to various activities of speech and hearing professionals, including counseling. Clinicians need to develop realistic expectations and goals. Sometimes change is immediate and other times it is relatively quick—but change also can be difficult and slow in other cases (Shipley & Wood, 1996). It is unreasonable to assume that all counselees can or will change dramatically in short periods of time. Clinicians need to view behavioral and attitudinal changes within incremental steps toward ultimate goals, realizing that there will be differences in the speed of change across individuals.

Providing Release and Support

Counseling can help people begin to understand and deal more effectively with situations they are experiencing. Webster (1968) comments that counseling

> *Can help parents to verbalize frankly about issues in their relationships and forces which motivate them, such as their needs, goals, and fears. Perhaps this is the most important thing that counseling offers parents: it provides them with a situation in which the clinician is willing for them to be themselves, to disclose their own thoughts and feelings; and to speak of their needs, anxieties, fears, joys, and successes.* (p. 334)

Providing support is a critical aspect of the counseling role. Patients need support, and so do family members, friends, and other caregivers. To achieve appropriate support, clinicians need to help counselees appreciate their strengths and understand their feelings and attitudes. Accomplishing this task requires empathy and an ability to relate to the needs of others.

The Role of Techniques

This book includes discussion about a variety of communication and interview techniques. However, the application of such techniques is no substitute for appropriate attitudes toward others. Counselors should never become so concerned about techniques and procedures that they lose perspective of sincere care for the people with whom they work (DeBlassie, 1976; Shipley & Wood, 1996).

Family Systems

The notion of family systems is that an individual lives within a unit, whether that unit is the immediate family, the extended family, or even something like foster care or an extended care facility. Any unit consists of sub-parts or sub-systems, which include: (1) relationships between family members; (2) relationships between the family and school and/ or the family and work; (3) the family's social support network (friends, other family members, church or other organizations); and (4) the legal system, social policy, and the public's attitudes that influence people with disabilities (adapted from Jones, 1993, p. 244).

As Jones notes, "like a pebble in water, a change in one system can cause a wave of changes in the others" (1993, p. 244). The notion of family systems is that all parts are tied together and, therefore, interdependent. Luterman (1991) considers the importance of family using the example of family therapists. As he comments:

> *For the family therapist there is no such thing as individual therapy; any time a change occurs in one member of the family, everybody in the family is impacted. Working in individual therapy with the identified patient in a dysfunctional family burdens the individual to become a change agent for the family. This is often too difficult a task for the patient, especially if it is a child. Family therapists find it much more efficacious to work at the family level.* (pp. 137-138)

Crais (1991) notes five basic themes of family-centered services:

- *Families are the constant in our client's lives, but service systems and individual professionals may only be sporadic;*
- *Families should be equal partners in the assessment and intervention process;*
- *Services should foster families' decision-making skills, while protecting their rights and wishes;*
- *Professionals need to recognize the individuality of clients and families and modify their own services to meet those needs; and*
- *Services must be delivered within a coordinated and "normalized" approach.* (p. 5)

Working with families is an established part of effective clinical practice in communicative disorders (see Hegde, 1993; Jones, 1993; Luterman,

1991; Rollin, 1987; Thornton, 1994; Schuyler & Rushmer, 1987; Webster & Ward, 1993; or others). However, family-centered services place greater emphasis on a partnership between the family and the professional rather than a more passive role by the family. Family systems are important to consider for effective practice because the individual and any changes desired do not occur in isolation; rather, they occur in relation to the family unit and in light of the various sub-systems affecting the individual and the family unit or units.

Groups

Some clinicians use a group model to provide certain counseling functions. This can be effective, useful, and a good use of time. It is also possible to accomplish certain things that are simply not possible in one-on-one interactions. Success in groups is related to several factors, including the specific needs of individuals in the group, the group's purposes, the members who make up the group, and the abilities of the clinician who is leading the group. Leith (1993) discusses three types of groups he has seen in speech therapy—the mob, therapy in groups, and group therapy. These categories are applicable to counseling activities.

- The *mob* is characterized by "chaos." The purpose is unclear and participants are often going in their own directions, often to the dismay of the clinician.
- *Therapy in groups* occurs when individuals work on different things but in a group setting, often waiting their turn to work on something specific to them. Essentially, individual work is being done but within a group of individuals.
- *Group therapy* implies interaction between members of a group. In effect, the group is involved with the treatment and progress that occurs.

Clearly the "mob" is unproductive and often frustrating to many of the participants. Such a group is out of control and accomplishes little, if anything. Therapy in a group can be effective in some settings because individuals work on particular areas of need. A true group therapy, with the possibility of some individualized work, is probably most beneficial with respect to counseling types of activities.

Goldberg (1993) suggests that groups in general have the following four basic functions:

1. To change speech and language behaviors
2. To provide a safe environment for practicing new speech and language behaviors
3. To provide opportunities for clients and caregivers to discuss the effects of a communicative disorder on their lives
4. To allow clinicians opportunities to observe, without interference, individuals' communicative behaviors

These are important functions that occur within well-designed group situations. Each of these functions has multiple possibilities. For example, communicative behavior can be changed in a number of ways, from helping someone practice fluent speech to having a new member observe what is possible. Those with similar communicative problems can communicate with others, release frustrations, or view techniques that work well for others. Clients or caregivers can discuss their situations, share concerns, learn from the successes of others, and many more. These are only a few of numerous other possibilities.

The basic principles discussed for sharing information and providing various counseling functions can be adapted for work in groups. Absolute prerequisites for effective group work are the same fundamentals of interviewing and counseling discussed in Chapter 1—having a purpose, a plan of action, and communicating clearly. Knowing what to address, and why, are important underpinnings of effective group practice. A group is approached a little differently, for example, when the purpose is to transmit certain information rather than to help clients share their feelings and concerns about a communicative disorder.

Often, groups are assembled by age (elementary, junior high, senior high, adult, and perhaps even older adult) and/or disorder type (aphasia, laryngectomy, fluency). Such groupings help expedite feelings of camaraderie and similarity among individuals. This is also helpful because, unlike the "therapy in groups" model noted earlier, members have a commonality of interest.

Support groups. Support groups exist for individuals with many speech and hearing problems—aphasia and post-stroke, stuttering, mental impairment, laryngectomy, to name just a few. Various support groups may be somewhat organized, or as "unorganized" as several people getting together for coffee from time to time. These groups are important and help serve several functions for individuals or caregivers involved with a communicative disorder (Atkins, 1994; Goldberg, 1993; Luterman, 1991; Rollin, 1987; Trace, 1993; Webster & Ward, 1993). They help members cope with their situations better, provide valuable interpersonal insights, help provide feedback about their "plight," and generally help reinforce and encourage members of the group (Goldberg, 1993).

Support groups are not counseling per se, but important activities occur. Among these, members meet others with similar circumstances, learn more about their own situations as well as those of others, acquire additional information about a disorder experienced, hear about the "trials and tribulations" of others, find out about possibilities that exist, and release frustrations and feelings with others who can relate directly to their experiences.

Some groups are established (or assisted) by clinicians; others are completely independent of any professional services. Thus, different groups function in a variety of ways. The points here are that support groups (1) meet important needs for many clients—they are frequently recommended for patients and caregivers; (2) assist clients and families in ways that clinicians often cannot; (3) are not counseling per se, and are not intended to replace the services we need to provide; and (4) are a valuable part of serving many patients' overall needs. They are not a threat or something that can or should be replaced, no matter how extensive and good counseling services are.

Role-Playing as a Technique

Role-playing—which involves the structured acting out or demonstrating of some behavior, or the roles specific behaviors play in the creation of problematic situations—is used in some clinical activities. For example, clinicians may have a patient who stutters practice fluent speech as if that person were talking with an employer, a loved one, someone in a store, and so forth. Webster (1968) describes role-playing as one method by which speech-language pathologists can work with parent groups.

One goal in role-playing might be to help people understand how specific feelings, attitudes, and behaviors are operating and then to identify alternative approaches for handling these problematic situations. The three basic components to role-playing are: (1) a leader who provides direction to the interaction, (2) a specific situation is acted out, and (3) there is then follow-up discussion.

Role-playing can help clients or caregivers explore and clarify their ideas and behavior, or attain valuable practice with some new skill. Role-playing can be useful in certain circumstances; however, Webster (1968) notes that it can have some disadvantages, particularly when focusing on feelings in groups. Role-playing can generate great fear or distress for individuals who have reservations or inhibitions about acting out their feelings. It can be difficult for some participants to reveal negative attitudes in front of a group. And, some participants may experience discomfort and separation when they find that their feelings differ dramatically from those of the rest of the group.

Examining Personal Abilities and the Effects of Counseling

Evaluating Personal Effectiveness

Stewart and Cash (1978) suggest that counselors can determine their general effectiveness by self-evaluation. These authors list six basic questions all counselors can ask themselves:

> 1. *Are you a good listener?*
> 2. *Do you have the patience necessary to deal with trying, time-consuming situations?*

3. Are you involved with a client or the client's problem?
4. Do you have a realistic view of your counseling skills, train-ing, and experiences?
5. Do you have a realistic view of what can and cannot be accomplished?
6. Do you have a sincere desire to help people without trying to play God? (p. 184)

These questions may be general and somewhat difficult to answer ob-jectively, but, they certainly are worth considering before and after any counseling interaction. Hackney and Cormier's (1994) Counseling Strat-egies Checklist (CSC) is a useful method for self-evaluation (see Appen-dix 7-B). Of course, the ultimate test of a clinician's effectiveness lies in whether the desired changes in feelings, attitudes, and behaviors occur with his or her counselees.

Evaluating Effects on Others

The observable effects of counseling efforts are the behavior and atti-tude changes that occur with counselees. Clinicians can evaluate the success of their efforts by asking whether a counselee followed specific suggestions, by counting the number of positive statements a counselee makes about a child or a spouse, by counting the number of "throat clears" in a prescribed time, or in many other ways. Charting the fre-quency and consistency of targeted attitudes or behaviors is an excel-lent method of examining treatment effects (see Hegde, 1993; Hegde & Davis, 1995; Mowrer, 1988; or others for information on baselining and charting). A counselor should take care to select evaluation methods that fit the goals of the treatment and that involve clearly defined, ob-servable behaviors or activities. If caregivers are being asked to apply behavioral principles, clinicians should carefully monitor the other party's use of the evaluation methods.

Signs of Difficulties

The idea of boundaries was addressed earlier in this chapter, and it also applies to personal effectiveness. Stone and Olswang (1989) comment that clinicians do not have to know precisely *why* something is a prob-lem to know that a problem exists. There are some " red flags" clinicians recognize when there are boundary problems, or they are "in over their heads"; the following are some of them:

- Interaction patterns are not satisfactory despite repeated attempts to cor-rect any problems.
- Counseling efforts fail to achieve desired results, or clients are getting worse.
- Clients become increasingly resistant to clinicians' efforts to help them.
- Clinicians are "getting pulled in deeper" to a client's problems or are sensing that they may not be able to resolve the problems.

- Patients respond in ways that differ from what clinicians are intending.
- Clinicians begin to develop feelings that are similar to, or more appropriate to, the client (e.g., anger, sadness, distress, remorse). (This is actually a psychological phenomenon called *countertransference*—clinicians begin to adopt the feelings of a particular client.)
- Clinicians become excessively worried or preoccupied with a case.
- Clinicians have persistent uncomfortable feelings about what is happening, even if these feelings or their source cannot be readily articulated. (Adapted from Stone & Olswang, 1989, p. 29.)

These guidelines are useful for helping to determine when there are problems within a counseling type of relationship. Note that any of these items is a signal of potential difficulties—this is not the type of list where a specified number of items checked "yes" indicates a problem, nor is it suggestive of the severity of a problem. Conscientious clinicians recognize such problems as early as possible so that appropriate actions can be started. There are a number of possible steps to take when identifying such a problem, including evaluating interactive methods, considering the topics of discussions and recommendations being made, consulting with a peer or supervisor, discussing the problem with the client or caregiver, and/or referring the client for more appropriate types of service. Exactly what is to be done will depend on the case, the extent of the problems, the relationship between the parties, the resources available, and the attitudes of people involved.

Concluding Comments

Clinicians frequently use the interviewing and counseling techniques described in this chapter and elsewhere in this book to bring about positive changes in the behavior, feelings, or attitudes of their clients. Behavioral counseling is a practical approach for speech-language pathologists and audiologists to use because it involves promoting change, skills in conditioning they already possess, and because it focuses on behavioral or attitudinal manifestations directly related to communicative disorders. Behavioral counseling is an effective approach for communicative disorders professionals because it allows for the close study of the effects of specific feelings and behaviors and the objective measurement of efforts to modify those attitudes or behaviors.

Cognitive approaches also are useful in speech-language pathology and audiology. These approaches allow the introduction and learning of new cognitive sets, which can promote tremendous progress and change within individuals. Often, clinicians use the best of both worlds—integrating behavioral and cognitive approaches together to promote optimal progress.

APPENDIX 7-A

EVALUATING INTERVIEWING AND COUNSELING SESSIONS WITH A CHECKLIST FORMAT

Check each item that applies.

1. *Length*
   _____ Adequate
   _____ Too short
   _____ Too long

2. *Amount of talking*
   _____ Counselor talked too much
   _____ Time well proportioned
   _____ Counselee talked too much

3. *Direction*
   _____ Counselee given every opportunity to express himself or herself
   _____ Counselee given some opportunity to express himself or herself
   _____ Counselee seldom given an opportunity to express himself or herself

4. *Amount of interest*
   _____ Monotonous, aimless, poor continuity
   _____ Some interesting spots
   _____ Interesting, well-directed, good continuity, climaxes

5. *Semantics*
   _____ Adapted to counselee
   _____ Sometimes inappropriate
   _____ Very inappropriate

6. *Responsibility*
   _____ Counselor assumed most of the responsibility
   _____ Counselor assumed some responsibility
   _____ Counselor gave full responsibility to counselee

7. *Depth*
   _____ Superficial
   _____ Some real problems discussed
   _____ Very adequate

8. *Interview controlled by*
   _____ Counselor
   _____ Counselee
   _____ Neither
   _____ Both

9. *Response to counselor*
   _____ Counselee responded easily
   _____ Counselee sometimes responded
   _____ Counselee resisted, would not respond

10. *Rapport*
    _____ High level of rapport maintained throughout
    _____ Rapport varied
    _____ Poor rapport

11. *Interaction and discussion between counselor and counselee*
    _____ A great deal
    _____ Some
    _____ Very little or none

12. *Did the counselor define the relationship between himself or herself and the counselee?*
    _____ Adequately
    _____ Somewhat
    _____ Poorly

13. *Did the counselor pave the way for follow-up?*
    _____ Adequately
    _____ Somewhat
    _____ Poorly

14. *Comments*

APPENDIX 7-B

COUNSELING STRATEGIES CHECKLIST

HOW TO USE THE COUNSELING STRATEGIES CHECKLIST (CSC).

Each item in the CSC is scored by circling the most appropriate response, either "Yes," "No," or "N.A." (not applicable). The items are worded so that desirable responses are "Yes" or "N.A." "No" is an undesirable response.

After the supervisor has observed and rated the interview, the two of you should sit down and review the ratings. Where noticeable deficiencies exist, you and the supervisor should identify a goal or goals that will remedy the problem. Beyond this, you should list two or three action steps that permit you to achieve the goal. After three or four more interviews, have the supervisor determine whether or not progress was evident.

PART I: Counselor Reinforcing Behavior (Nonverbal)

1. The counselor maintained eye contact with the client.
   Yes   No   N.A.

2. The counselor displayed several different facial expressions during the interview.
   Yes   No   N.A.

3. The counselor's facial expressions reflected the mood of the client.
   Yes   No   N.A.

4. The counselor often responded to the client with facial animation and alertness.
   Yes   No   N.A.

5. The counselor displayed intermittent head movements (up-down, side-to-side).
   Yes   No   N.A.

6. The counselor refrained from head nodding when the client did not pursue goal-directed topics.
   Yes   No   N.A.

7. The counselor demonstrated a relaxed body position.
   Yes   No   N.A.

8. The counselor leaned forward as a means of encouraging the client to engage in some goal-directed behavior.
   Yes   No   N.A.

9. The counselor demonstrated some variation in voice pitch when talking.
   Yes   No   N.A.

10. The counselor's voice was easily heard by the client.
    Yes   No   N.A.

Source: From Harold Hackney and Sherry Cormier, *Counseling Strategies and Interventions* (4th ed.), pp. 192-200. Copyright 1994 and reprinted by permission of Allyn and Bacon, Boston, MA.

11. The counselor used intermittent one-word vocalizations ("mm-hmm") to reinforce the client's demonstration of goal-directed topics or behaviors.
Yes   No   N.A.

Counselor Reinforcing Behavior (Verbal)

12. The counselor usually spoke slowly enough so that each word was easily understood.
Yes   No   N.A.

13. A majority (60 percent or more) of the counselor's responses could be categorized as complete sentences rather than monosyllabic phrases.
Yes   No   N.A.

14. The counselor's verbal statements were concise and to the point.
Yes   No   N.A.

15. The counselor refrained from repetition in verbal statements.
Yes   No   N.A.

16. The counselor made verbal comments that pursued the topic introduced by the client.
Yes   No   N.A.

17. The subject of the counselor's verbal statements usually referred to the client, either by name or the second-person pronoun, "you."
Yes   No   N.A.

18. A clear and sensible progression of topics was evident in the counselor's verbal behavior; the counselor avoided rambling.
Yes   No   N.A.

PART II: Opening Interview

1. In the first part of the interview, the counselor used several different nonverbal gestures (smiling, head nodding, hand movement, etc.) to help put the client at ease.
Yes   No   N.A.

2. In starting the interview, the counselor remained silent or invited the client to talk about whatever he or she wanted, thus leaving the selection of initial topic up to the client.
Yes   No   N.A.

3. After the first five minutes of the interview, the counselor refrained from encouraging social conversation.
Yes   No   N.A.

4. After the first topic of discussion was exhausted, the counselor remained silent until the client identified a new topic.
Yes   No   N.A.

5. The counselor provided structure (information about nature, purposes of counseling, time limits, etc.) when the client indicated uncertainty about the interview.
Yes   No   N.A.

6. In beginning the initial interview, the counselor used at least one of the following structuring procedures:
    a. Provided information about taping and/or observation
    b. Commented on confidentiality
    c. Made remarks about the counselor's role and purpose of the interview
    d. Discussed with the client his or her expectations about counseling
    Yes   No   N.A.

PART III: Termination of the Interview

1. The counselor informed the client before terminating that the interview was almost over.
   Yes   No   N.A.

2. The counselor refrained from introducing new material (a different topic) at the termination phase of the interview.
   Yes   No   N.A.

3. The counselor discouraged the client from pursuing new topics within the last five minutes of the interview by avoiding asking for further information about it.
   Yes   No   N.A.

4. Only one attempt to terminate the interview was required before the termination was actually completed.
   Yes   No   N.A.

5. The counselor initiated the termination of the interview through use of some closing strategy such as acknowledgment of time limits and/or summarization (by self or client).
   Yes   No   N.A.

6. At the end of the interview, the counselor offered the client an opportunity to return for another interview.
   Yes   No   N.A.

PART IV: Goal Setting

1. The counselor asked the client to identify some of the conditions surrounding the occurrence of the client's problem ("when do you feel _____ ?").
   Yes   No   N.A.

2. The counselor asked the client to identify some of the consequences resulting from the client's behavior ("What happens when you _____ ?").
   Yes   No   N.A.

3. The counselor asked the client to state how he or she would like to change his or her behavior ("How would you like for things to be different?").
   Yes   No   N.A.

4. The counselor and client decided together on counseling goals.
   Yes   No   N.A.

5. The goals set in the interview were specific and observable.
   Yes   No   N.A.

6. The counselor asked the client to orally state a commitment to work for goal achievement.
   Yes   No   N.A.

7. If the client appeared resistant or unconcerned about achieving change, the counselor discussed this with the client.
   Yes   No   N.A.

8. The counselor asked the client to specify at least one action step he or she might take toward his or her goal.
   Yes   No   N.A.

9. The counselor suggested alternatives available to the client.
   Yes   No   N.A.

10. The counselor helped the client to develop action steps for goal attainment.
    Yes   No   N.A.

11. Action steps designated by counselor and client were specific and realistic in scope.
    Yes   No   N.A.

12. The counselor provided an opportunity within the interview for the client to practice or rehearse the action step.
    Yes   No   N.A.

13. The counselor provided feedback to the client concerning the execution of the action step.
    Yes   No   N.A.

14. The counselor encouraged the client to observe and evaluate the progress and outcomes of action steps taken outside the interview.
    Yes   No   N.A.

PART V: Counselor Discrimination

1. The counselor's responses were usually directed toward the most important component of each of the client's communications.
   Yes   No   N.A.

2. The counselor followed client topic changes by responding to the primary cognitive or affective idea, reflecting a common theme in each communication.
   Yes   No   N.A.

3. The counselor usually identified and responded to the feelings of the client.
   Yes   No   N.A.

4. The counselor usually identified and responded to the behaviors of the client.
   Yes   No   N.A.

5. The counselor verbally acknowledged several (at least two) nonverbal affect cues.
   Yes   No   N.A.

6. The counselor encouraged the client to talk about his or her feelings.
   Yes   No   N.A.

7. The counselor encouraged the client to identify and evaluate his or her actions.
   Yes   No   N.A.

8. The counselor discouraged the client from making and accepting excuses (rationalization) for his or her behavior.
   Yes   No   N.A.

9. The counselor asked questions that the client could not answer in a "yes" or "no" fashion (typically beginning with words such as how, what, when, where, who, etc.).
   Yes   No   N.A.

10. Several times (at least two) the counselor confronted the client with a discrepancy present in the client's communication and/or behavior.
    Yes   No   N.A.

11. Several times (at least two) the counselor used responses that supported or reinforced something the client said or did.
    Yes   No   N.A.

12. The counselor used several (at least two) responses that suggested a course of action the client had the potential for completing in the future.
    Yes   No   N.A.

13. Sometimes the counselor restated or clarified the client's previous communication.
    Yes   No   N.A.

14. The counselor used several (at least two) responses that summarized ambivalent and conflicting feelings of the client.
    Yes   No   N.A.

15. The counselor encouraged discussion of negative feelings (anger, fear) expressed by the client.
    Yes   No   N.A.

15. Several times (at least two) the counselor suggested how the client might feel about a particular topic.
    Yes   No   N.A.

PART VI: The Process of Relating

1. The counselor made statements that reflected the client's feelings.
   Yes   No   N.A.

2. The counselor responded to the core of a long and ambivalent client statement.
   Yes   No   N.A.

3. The counselor verbally stated his or her desire and/or intent to understand.
   Yes   No   N.A.

4. The counselor made verbal statements that the client reaffirmed without qualifying or changing the counselor's previous response.
   Yes   No   N.A.

5. The counselor made attempts to verbally communicate his or her understanding of the client that elicited an affirmative client response ("Yes, that's exactly right," and so forth).
   Yes   No   N.A.

6. The counselor reflected the client's feelings at the same or a greater level of intensity than originally expressed by the client.
   Yes   No   N.A.

7. In communicating understanding of the client's feelings, the counselor verbalized the anticipation present in the client's communication (i.e., what the client would like to do or how the client would like to be).
   Yes   No   N.A.

8. The counselor frowned when failing to understand what the client was saying.
   Yes   No   N.A.

9. The counselor verbalized personal confusion or misunderstanding to the client.
   Yes   No   N.A.

10. The counselor nodded when agreeing with or encouraging the client.
    Yes   No   N.A.

11. When the counselor's nonverbal behavior suggested that he or she was uncertain or disagreeing, the counselor verbally acknowledged this to the client.
    Yes   No   N.A.

12. The counselor answered directly when the client asked about his or her opinion or reaction.
    Yes   No   N.A.

13. The counselor encouraged discussion of statements made by the client that challenged the counselor's knowledge and beliefs.
    Yes   No   N.A.

14. Several times (at least twice) the counselor shared his or her own feelings with the client.
    Yes   No   N.A.

15. At least one time during the interview the counselor provided specific feedback to the client.
    Yes   No   N.A.

16. The counselor encouraged the client to identify and discuss his or her feelings concerning the counselor and the interview.
    Yes   No   N.A.

17. The counselor voluntarily shared his or her feelings about the client and the counseling relationship.
    Yes   No   N.A.

18. The counselor expressed reactions about the client's strengths and/or potential.

Yes   No   N.A.

19. The counselor made responses that reflected his or her liking and appreciation of the client.

Yes   No   N.A.

Working with Linguistically and Culturally Diverse Clients

CELESTE ROSEBERRY-McKIBBIN

Like a kaleidoscope that is continually changing colors, the ethnic and linguistic composition of U.S. society is becoming more and more richly diverse. As Montgomery and Herer (1994) state, we live in "an increasingly multicultural society, one that is more linguistically diverse; a whiter, older society and younger, browner one" (p. 131). Indeed, there is an increasing number of linguistically and culturally diverse (LCD) individuals in the United States (Fitzgerald, 1995).

This increasing diversity comes primarily from changes in immigration trends and birth rates. In 1820, 92% of immigrants were European; in 1990, 7% of immigrants were from European backgrounds (U.S. Bureau of the Census, 1992). During the 1980s, the Asian/Pacific Islander population increased by 95%, the Hispanic population increased by 52%, the African American population increased by 13%, and the non-Hispanic whites increased by 4% (Gall & Gall, 1993). The European American birth rate in the United States has been declining since 1964 (Tidwell, Kuumba, Jones, & Watson, 1993). By the year 2005, whites will have a 0.8% population decrease (Horton & Smith, 1993), and during the twenty-first century, ethnic and racial minorities will outnumber whites for the first time (Henry, 1990).

It is estimated that at least one third of school children in the United States will be either Asian, African American, Hispanic, or native American in the year 2000 (Lane & Molyneaux, 1992). Demographers believe that by the year 2020, one out of every three persons in the United States will be from what is now referred to as a "minority group" (Sobol, 1990). The American Speech-Language-Hearing Association (ASHA, 1988, as cited in Larson & McKinley, 1995) estimates that in the year 2000, seven million persons of minority origin will have communicative disorders that warrant intervention. Statistics indicate that the majority of speech-language pathologists are Anglo-European, monolingual English speakers. According to ASHA (1992), only 3.7% of ASHA's members and certificate holders identified themselves as black, Hispanic, Asian, or Native American. Thankfully this is changing, but the changes are slow.

As clinicians hone their skills in interviewing and counseling, these skills must necessarily include the ability to relate to clients and families from LCD backgrounds whose needs and experiences differ from those of the dominant U.S. culture. Accordingly, the overall purpose of this chapter is to alert readers to ideas that will increase their confidence and skill when dealing with clients from diverse backgrounds. Readers are strongly encouraged to read other sources in greater depth to enhance and expand on the points that are introduced and summarized in this chapter.

Dr. Shipley has talked about various multiculturally related implications in various places throughout this book. Some of the information in this chapter is also seen or alluded to in other places, and readers will notice several instances of repetition. The reason that important points are reiterated here is to ensure that these points don't just "fade into the woodwork," so to speak. In our increasingly multicultural society, clinicians must be knowledgeable about and sensitive to important issues in serving diverse clients. This chapter attempts to ensure that important issues are discussed and reinforced—repetition is the mother of skill!

Variables Influencing Individuals from Different Cultures

Most clinicians are aware of the importance of not stereotyping individuals from particular cultural groups. Instead of viewing various cultural groups as homogeneous and monolithic, Hanson (1992) recommends that clinicians take a situational and transactional approach in which individual clients and families are recognized as having unique characteristics and needs. Culture is dynamic (Green & Perlman, 1995), and clinicians will relate to their clients more skillfully if they realize that each individual within a cultural group is influenced by a number of variables (Roseberry-McKibbin, 1995). Linguistically and culturally diverse values, behavior, and utilization of services are all heavily impacted by characteristics that make each client unique. Clinicians who serve these diverse clients must take these characteristics into account so that clients will be seen as individuals and valued as such, not just seen as members of a certain homogeneous group. Some of the variables to consider are addressed in the following sections.

Generational Membership

Clinicians should ascertain whether certain clients are first-, second-, or third-generation members of the country of current residence, or whether their family has resided in the country even longer. Generational membership may make a difference in clients' openness to and belief in the efficacy of and necessity for our services.

Length of Residence

Clients may be long-term residents of an area with concomitant support systems. Or, they may be new residents with little or no support who will need greater assistance from professionals.

Degree of Adaptation to Mainstream Culture

There are different ways in which diverse clients, especially refugees and immigrants, may adapt to U.S. culture. Some groups may adapt by integrating into mainstream cultural life more fully than others who desire to maintain separateness. Professionals should attempt to discover how individual clients and families have chosen to adapt to mainstream culture, because the degree of adaptation can affect clients' receptivity toward speech, language, and hearing services. Cheng and Butler (1993) describe the following various degrees of adaptation:

- *Reaffirmation*—there are efforts to revive native cultural traditions. Persons may reject the majority culture.
- *Synthesis*—there is a selective combination of cultural aspects of both cultures.
- *Withdrawal*—there is a rejection of both cultures because they conflict; persons do not commit to either culture.
- *Compensatory adaptation*—individuals thoroughly mainstream into the new culture; they reject and avoid identifying with their home culture.
- *Biculturalism*—there is full involvement with both cultures; persons must be able to make smooth transitions between both cultures.
- *Constructive marginality*—there is a tentative acceptance of two cultures; individuals do not fully integrate into either one.

Again, clients' degree of adaptation may impact on the provision of services for communicative disorders.

Socioeconomic Status and Upward Mobility

Increasingly, on our shrinking globe, individuals are viewed not so much on the basis of homogeneous cultural categories, but along lines of social class (Walton, 1995). Socioeconomic status has considerable impact on who LCD clients are, and it can affect issues like clients' acceptance of Western medicine, understanding of the need for and nature of special education or rehabilitation, and so forth. Socioeconomic status also greatly impacts clients' ability to afford therapy in settings where patients are charged for services.

Educational Level

Highly educated clients of any cultural background may respond differently in counseling and interviewing situations than clients who have not had the benefit of formal education. For less-educated clients, interviewing or counseling may be unfamiliar concepts and thus discomforting events. Clients who have little or no formal education may also have difficulty with written documentation, meetings with groups of professionals, and with carrying out written instructions that are provided.

Urban or Rural Background

Clients (especially immigrants or refugees) from rural backgrounds may feel more intimidated by large and/or formal settings, paperwork, and technology than clients from urban backgrounds (Arambula, 1992). This may impact clients' willingness to participate in rehabilitation involving surgery, therapy, medicine, or assistive devices such as motorized wheelchairs. It may also cause them to feel uncomfortable with (and thus avoid) large, complicated buildings such as medical centers.

Age and Gender

Among many cultures, there are strong social and role expectation lines between men and women, and the old and young. Each group has its various roles and accompanying expectations.

Languages Spoken

Speech, language, and hearing services will be impacted by clients' language status. For example, clients may be monolingual speakers of their primary language, fluent speakers of English, or they may demonstrate language skills on a large continuum of proficiency in between these two points.

Impact of Immigrant/Refugee Status on Multicultural Clients

Clinicians are increasingly working with multicultural clients who are of immigrant or refugee status. It is important to understand the impact of immigrant/refugee status on clients and their families and the possible effects on interviewing, counseling, and accompanying assessment and treatment efforts.

An *immigrant* is defined as a person who comes to a country to take up permanent residence. A *refugee* is someone who flees to a new country or power for safety or to escape danger or persecution (*Merriam-Webster Collegiate Dictionary,* 1993). There is enormous diversity among immigrants and refugees; they represent every echelon of society, from great wealth and privilege to poverty and illiteracy. They speak English in varying degrees, and experience varying levels of acculturation to U.S. life.

Clinicians must look at factors that tend to result in a higher level of acculturation. Immigrants and refugees who have achieved a high level of acculturation are frequently more comfortable with speech-language-hearing services than those who have a lower level of acculturation. Factors that tend to result in higher levels of acculturation are: urban (as opposed to rural) origin, higher socioeconomic status, a relatively high level of formal education, immigration to the United States at an early age, birth into a family that has been in the new country for at least several years, limited migration back and forth to the country of origin, and extensive contact with people outside the family and/or ethnic network (Leslie, 1992; Randall-David, 1989). Immigrants and refugees with lower levels of acculturation may experience specific challenges which clinicians need to consider. These challenges impact service delivery to many clients who were born in another country.

Many refugees have witnessed and/or endured oppressive and traumatic experiences—persecution, disease, atrocities, forced labor, death of or separation from family members, starvation, and being uprooted. These types of problems can result in post-traumatic stress disorders, health problems, and many other negative sequelae (Kinzie, Sack, Angell, Clarke, & Ben, 1989). Clients who have undergone these types of experiences may need additional emotional support and counseling activities. A psychologist or other support personnel may be necessary for some clients.

Family life in the United States is often very different from that experienced in the country of origin. Older students—especially teenagers—may experience substantial difficulties because schools are considerably different from schools in their home country. U.S. schools tend to be more liberal and less formal than schools in many other countries, and this is often associated with adjustment difficulties for students and parents. School in the United States is compulsory for immigrant children who arrive in their teenage years; in some countries, schooling is not required beyond 12 or 13 years of age. Compulsory school attendance may cause conflict between laws and cultural traditions. Some parents may discourage children from going to school, feeling that school attendance is selfish and that the children should be involved in helping support the family rather than "indulging" in continuing education (Cheng & Ima, 1989).

Another stress for many immigrant and refugee families is experiencing poverty. Many individuals were well-paid, highly respected professionals in their home lands. They encounter new barriers because of their heavy accents, or because their professional training is not accepted in the new land. Some people were dentists, lawyers, and architects in their native countries, but they may be working as custodians or secretaries in the new country, causing adjustment problems. Clinicians must be sensitive to this—the taxi driver sitting in their office today may have been a surgeon or accountant in his or her home country. Clinicians must not assume that a lack of formal education is necessarily related to a client's current job.

Many cultures have definite lines of social status related to age, gender, and place in the family. In many countries, elders (parents and grandparents) are accorded great respect and are obeyed because they are authority figures. When families come to the United States, where youth is venerated and elders are often disrespected, many families are caught in great conflicts. Elders who have had absolute authority often find that their children no longer exhibit automatic, unquestioning obedience. Many elders feel like they have lost their power and dignity. Elders may want young people to maintain the "traditional" cultural ways, and the young people want to adopt the values, customs, and lifestyles of the new culture.

Children and youth often learn English more quickly than their elders and become family spokespersons, further usurping elders' traditional roles as authority figures (Rick & Forward, 1992). Children may want to marry an individual from the new culture instead of someone from their home culture and/or religious groups—elders may vehemently disagree with this and look on marriage to an "outsider" as a great personal tragedy for the family. For example, I have worked with university students who would not consider marrying outside their cultural group because of the heartbreak it would bring to their families. However, other individuals would consider such choices.

In some families, marital relationships may become disharmonious if women who have traditionally stayed home and obeyed their husbands start working outside the home to earn money for the family (Rick & Forward, 1992). Also, when mothers who have stayed at home begin working long hours outside the home to survive financially, children may go unsupervised and feel a loss of attention. This can lead to discipline problems, truancy, and even gang membership. Life in the United States, with its dual-income households and emphasis on independence, tends to fragment some families who have traditionally been interdependent and relied on each other to meet most needs (Sharifzadeh, 1992).

Another stress for many immigrant and refugee families is the general feeling among many in the public that immigrants are causing many social and economic problems that threaten current and future mainstream culture (Hayes-Bautista, Hurtado, Valdez, & Hernandez, 1992). There is considerable fear leading to legislative proposals to stem the flow of new immigrants (Leslie, 1992). Clinicians who work with immigrants and refugees must make sure they do not hold biases that could negatively impact their clinical effectiveness, including interviewing and counseling activities.

Certain health problems may affect immigrants and refugees. For example, I have worked with some Vietnamese clients who were born during the fall of Saigon, malnutrition was rampant and prenatal care was practically nonexistent at that time. Subsequent problems in school often stem from maternal illness and lack of nutrition in utero. In other situations, some refugees who spent considerable time in refugee camps had little or no medical care, impacting children's speech and language development, adults' predisposition toward strokes, and so forth.

Clinicians who work with immigrant and refugee clients need to be especially sensitive to these types of factors, and consider how they may impact interviewing and counseling activities. An increased awareness of these factors assists clinicians in being supportive, understanding, and more effective.

Values, Assumptions, and Linguistically and Culturally Diverse Clients

Many readers of this book are from mainstream U.S. backgrounds where certain values and assumptions exist—many of them unconsciously. Although clinicians recognize that their own value systems are important and intrinsic parts of their being, they cannot optimally serve LCD populations without becoming consciously aware of their own values and assumptions—and how they unconsciously may be imposing these values onto their clients.

Clinicians who come from a mainstream background of the dominant culture must carefully examine their own assumptions and values. They must make sure they do not communicate that clients are wrong or inferior for believing differently about issues such as the necessity of therapy, family participation in therapy, and so forth. The tendency to see one's own culture as correct, natural, and superior to another culture is called *ethnocentrism* (Lane & Molyneaux, 1992). Clinicians can successfully work with multicultural families by avoiding ethnocentrism, respecting these families' beliefs, cultural mores, and working with families to find paths that are culturally acceptable and are best for individual clients' welfare.

The following sections summarize some commonly held values and assumptions among persons of mainstream backgrounds. Awareness of these values and assumptions helps clinicians to avoid letting them hinder effectiveness in working with diverse clients.

Time

Assumption—"Punctuality is important and is an intrinsic part of a professional relationship based on mutual respect."

United States culture is monochronic—adherence to schedules and timeliness is very important. Punctuality is essential. Some cultures are *polychronic;* that is, members of those cultures stress completion of transactions and involvement of people rather than strict adherence to schedules (Reyes, 1994). Time is very "elastic" and punctuality is not particularly important in polychronic cultures. For example, in Micronesia, families might arrive 15 to 30 minutes after appointments are to begin (Hammer, 1994). In the Philippines, if an event is scheduled for 11:00, it might not actually begin until 11:45 or 12:00. Promptness within some cultures is rarely a priority. Clinicians must be understanding of this; on the other hand, clinicians should also communicate to clients that if they are late and the clinician's schedule is full, clients may miss their appointment completely. Clear communication is imperative, as families may be offended if they arrive 30 minutes late and find that they must be rescheduled because the next meeting has already started.

Beginning an Interaction

Assumption—"In professional situations such as meetings, it is important to 'get down to business' as quickly and efficiently as possible."

Among most mainstream U.S. people, getting to the point quickly is valued. However, this may offend some culturally diverse families. In the Hispanic culture, for example, business conversations are often preceded by lengthy chatting about topics unrelated to the purpose of the meeting (Larson & McKinley, 1995). Zuniga (1992) states that professionals who work with Hispanic families should engage in *platicando*—leisurely and friendly interaction that sets the stage for work to occur. Among many Japanese, informal socializing precedes "cutting to the chase"; those who get right down to business are perceived as rude and abrupt. Clinicians must determine what style is most comfortable for each client.

Formality Versus Informality

> *Assumption*—"Informality and social equality are the ultimate goals in all interactions between professionals and clients."

In some cultures, social status and hierarchy are very important. For example, many Japanese find it awkward and unbecoming if people do not interact according to status expectations. Social roles are clearly delineated along the lines of relative status, and people are expected to behave accordingly with appropriate courtesy and deference. In the Japanese language, there are approximately 100 words for "I" and "me." The form used depends on many variables such as the speaker's age and gender, the formality of the occasion, and the interlocutors' relative status (Cheng, 1987).

In many cultures, such as the African American and Asian cultures, politeness and the use of titles are considered common courtesy (Chan, 1992a; Tiegerman-Farber, 1995). Among Hispanics, respect for individuals with advanced age and experience is commonly connoted by using "Usted" (formal "you") rather than "tu" (informal or familiar "you") (Langdon, 1992). Persons from some cultures might be offended if clinicians call them by their first names, and they would consider it highly inappropriate to call clinicians by their first names. Within the confines of maintaining confidentiality, it is best for clinicians to ask interpreters or others who know a family what would be most appropriate for each particular situation. If clinicians are unsure, it is best to err on the side of being more formal.

Directness

> *Assumption*—"Frankness, openness, and honest discussion of situations and feelings is important."

Although most people believe that talking indirectly shows powerlessness and insecurity, indirectness is the norm in many cultures. For example, among most Japanese, social norms dictate that harmony should be maintained, conflict should be avoided, and that almost no one says "no" out in public (Tannen, 1994). Among many Asians, indirect communication styles are the norm (Chan, 1992a). Clinicians must be careful, because what the mainstream population considers direct and open communication may be perceived as offensively blunt by some clients.

Gender

> *Assumption*—"The gender of the clinician and the client is not important; the clinician's competence is the most important variable."

Ideally this is true, but for some ethnic groups, the clinician's gender is an important variable. For example, among some cultures and religious groups, it is considered highly offensive for a female clinician to ask direct questions of a male client (Culatta & Goldberg, 1995). Likewise, in other groups, a male clinician would never be allowed alone in a room, unsupervised, with a female client. As another example, most Middle Eastern women would feel deep discomfort discussing, in an information-getting interview situation, personal issues such as childbirth with a male clinician (Sharifzadeh, 1992). Opposite-sex clinicians would not be allowed to work with some Hindus (Nellum-Davis, 1993). In some Iraqi families, women cannot leave the house without permission of their husbands (Buell, 1985); thus, it may be difficult for some Iraqi men to work with "liberated" female professionals. These "gender lines" are difficult for many clinicians who have been taught that gender should not matter in professional situations. But, to be optimally effective, clinicians need to provide interactional situations for clients that are comfortable and that will elicit the most optimal cooperation and communication possible.

Age

Assumption—"The age of a clinician, relative to the client, is unimportant as long as the clinician is competent."

In many cultures—for example, Middle Eastern, Native American, Asian, and Hispanic—age is accompanied by increased respect. The older person is the one to be respected and whose opinions are sought. Conversely, young people are seen as having less wisdom and, thus, are less deserving of respect. Young clinicians may want to work in concert with an older professional or interpreter in situations where youth is a barrier to effective service.

Written Documentation

Assumption—"Written documentation is a necessary and intrinsic part of professionals' interactions with clients and families."

Some limited- or non-English proficient families may feel intimidated by the presence of written forms. Paperwork is not a part of interactions in many cultures, and in some cultures, signatures are only required for significant life events such as births or deaths (Cheng & Hammer, 1992). In other cultures, there is an oral tradition with no tradition of literacy. The Southeast Asian Hmong, for example, had no written language until recent years (Ima & Cheng, 1989). Some native American groups have only recently created systems for writing down information (Bouty, 1992). Professionals in these situations should rely more on oral than written communication. In situations where paperwork is necessary, it is sometimes best if an interpreter is present to thoroughly explain the nature of and the need for it.

Nature of Disabilities

> *Assumption*—"Speech and language therapy are usually necessary even if the client does not have an overt physical handicap."

In the United States, clinicians frequently treat clients for "invisible handicaps"—specific language impairment, cognitive impairment, learning disability, stuttering, or voice disorders, for example. In some cultures, however, such as the Hispanic and Asian cultures, it is believed that only physical disabilities merit treatment (Matsuda, 1989). Some Asian clients believe that persons with speech disorders and no accompanying overt physical impairment can improve if they "try hard." These clients are less apt to seek treatment for a stuttering child, for instance, because they believe the child is not trying hard enough (Bebout & Arthur, 1992).

I recall working with two Hmong elementary-aged boys who had chronically low, hoarse voices characterized by pitch and phonation breaks. At my request, an interpreter called the home to speak with the parents about taking the boys to an ear, nose, and throat physician for an evaluation of the boys' vocal folds so that appropriate therapy could be provided. The interpreter told me later that, although the parents said they would follow through, he was not sure they would actually do this because only overt and visible physical disabilities merit intervention in the Hmong culture.

Intervention and Independence

> *Assumption*—"Rehabilitation is usually necessary because the goal for all individuals, including those with speech and language impairments, is to be as independent as possible."

According to Wallace (1993), some groups believe that a person experiencing a difficulty or impairment

> *needs to experience the challenges associated with the illness rather than receive treatment to overcome the illness . . . for [other] cultures . . . tradition indicates that the ill person is to be "taken care of" rather than rehabilitated back to independency. In such instances, requiring the patient to attend rehabilitation services to learn to function independently would be considered disrespectful and would cause great shame to the family.* (p. 248)

Among some Asians, rehabilitation for the impaired individual might bring great shame to the whole family because they believe that caring for this individual is their responsibility (Chan, 1992a). Among some Hispanics, friends and family may indulge children with impairments. These children may not be expected to actively participate in their own care and treatment (National Coalition of Hispanic Health and Human Services Organization, 1988). In cases such as these, a clinician's efforts

to direct families toward rehabilitation may be viewed as being culturally insensitive and could be counterproductive.

Western Intervention

Assumption—"When clients display speech-language disabilities,
Western forms of intervention are the most effective and appropriate."

When clients exhibit speech, language, or hearing disabilities, clinicians
often recommend therapy. They may also recommend that clients seek
out physicians who may then prescribe surgery, medications, physical
therapy, or other rehabilitative services or assistive devices. Sometimes
professionals discover to their chagrin that families of clients with communicative disorders, instead, are using what would be considered "non-
traditional" forms of healing such as prayer, roots, herbs, massage, and
witch doctors or medicine persons. Most Buddhist Laotians, for example,
believe that every human being has 32 souls; when a person is sick, a
sorcerer performs the ritual of Baci to call back the souls of the sick
person in order to help the person recover (Cheng, 1991). Some Native
American families, when a family member has an illness or disability,
conduct traditional ceremonies before they become involved in programs recommended by service providers (Joe & Malach, 1992). Many
members of the Hmong culture do not want surgical intervention because they believe that spirits in the patient's body may leave (Cheng &
Hammer, 1992).

In other situations, persons whose customs include holistic care,
folk medicine, and prayer may feel they are not being treated respectfully by medical and rehabilitation personnel, and thus, may not follow
their recommendations. Other groups, such as some Asians and Pacific
Islanders, view severely disabling conditions with great stigma. They
may believe that a child's disability represents God's punishment for
sins (Mokuau & Tauili'ili, 1992), and may thus be reluctant to seek out
services because they want to "save face" (Allen, McNeill, & Schmidt,
1992; Chan, 1992a). Clinicians would do best to work with—not against—
healers, forms of healing, and beliefs that are appropriate to clients'
cultures (Maestas & Erickson, 1992; Wallace, 1993).

Family Participation

Assumption—"When a particular client is receiving rehabilitative
services or therapy, the family must be as active as possible in collaboration with the clinician."

All clinicians recognize the importance of including families in any interviewing, counseling, and assessment or treatment; many experts

emphasize the need for clinician-family collaboration (Lund & Duchan, 1993; Larson & McKinley, 1995; Tiegerman-Farber, 1995). Clinicians frequently counsel families that they need to be actively involved in the treatment or rehabilitation process for a family member with a speech, language, or hearing disorder. However, in some cultures, the professional or agency is supposed to "take care of" the client; families may be uncomfortable with or unprepared for the amount or type of family participation expected of them (Bondurant-Utz, 1994). Families may be taken by surprise when professionals expect them to be actively involved, for example, in a child's special education or an elderly person's rehabilitation after a stroke. Lynch and Hanson (1992b) give the example of a multicultural mother of a disabled child who was uncomfortable being asked for her thoughts about her child's service needs. To this mother, "it was inappropriate for parents to be questioned about services because 'that was the job of the professionals to decide'" (p. 363).

Control of Destiny

Assumption—"Individuals have control over their own destinies."

Many people are very deterministic; that is, they believe they have a great deal of personal control over their futures and what happens to them. In the paradigm of "self-contained individualism," which characterizes most of the U.S. mainstream, professionals expect that clients will "aspire toward internal control and an exercise of personal responsibility in their own lives" (Dana, 1993, p. 16). But in some cultures, which might be wrongly labeled as "passive," individuals may believe that fate or the gods shape their destinies. For example, Cheng (1989) notes that Taoism, practiced by many Chinese:

> *Promotes passivity, and those who practice it may display a sense of fatalism . . . resulting in resignation and inaction. This basic principle of nonintervention may have a deleterious effect when parents are asked to approve intervention for remediation of language or learning disorders.* (p. 183)

Many Native Americans believe in accepting circumstances and taking life as it comes (Joe & Malach, 1992), and may seem as though they are too passive in situations where treatment is needed for a family member. In counseling situations, clinicians need to strike a delicate balance between addressing some clients' beliefs (e.g., that rehabilitation and/or therapy are not needed because the disability is the will of God or fate) and encouraging families to actively explore as many therapy/rehabilitation options as possible.

Language in the Home

> *Assumption*—"Families who speak other languages at home need to speak English to their children so that the children will learn English."

In some interviewing and counseling situations, clinicians have been known to recommend that parents who speak broken English need to speak English, rather than their primary language, to their children. This pernicious and oft-given advice has deleterious impacts on children's language development and family communication in general (ASHA, 1995a; Kayser, 1993; Fillmore, 1993). Family members should speak to one another in the language they are the most comfortable using (Ima & Cheng, 1989). It is the quality of the interaction, not the language of the interaction, that is the key for children's development. Professionals should emphasize to parents that being bilingual is positive and that speaking two or more languages is a great asset in today's world.

Counseling Individuals

> *Assumption*—"Counseling individuals in isolation can be quite effective."

U.S. culture has been termed a "low-context culture" where an emphasis is placed on the role of the individual. However, many clients come from cultures where the individual is recognized primarily as a member of a group, not as an individual entity (Joe & Malach, 1992; Westby & Rouse, 1985). As Dana (1993) states:

> *The relentless focus on the self provided by most existing services may be alien and disquieting to persons with cultural values that define the self only in concert with others and perceive autonomy and individualism as undesirable or even unnecessary.* (p. 16)

In many situations, it is imperative for clinicians to involve the whole family in interviewing and counseling situations, not just individual members. Decision making, in many cultures, involves the whole family, including extended family members.

Along this line, it may be important to help families get support from other members of their culture. Many families, especially newly arrived immigrants and refugees, feel isolated. Support groups can be highly effective for some of these families (Ruiz, 1991). Professionals can consider recommending local churches, community centers, and other resources when appropriate. For example, several experts state that many African Americans have strong ties with the church (Hanline & Daley, 1992; Terrell & Terrell 1993; Willis, 1992). It might be appropriate for clinicians to use religious organizations as allies in intervention when working with some African American clients (Randall-David, 1989). Clinicians should try to recommend support systems that are appropriate for each family.

Communicating Effectively When Interviewing and Counseling

Clients come into interviewing and counseling situations with varying degrees of proficiency in the English language. This can present certain challenges for effective communication between clinicians and clients or families. The following suggestions are useful for clinicians to implement with clients who are experiencing difficulties communicating in English.

Loudness

Do not increase the volume of your voice. Clients (with the exception of the hearing impaired) do not need clinicians to shout at them or speak in loud tones. It is shocking to see how many clinicians speak loudly to individuals whose English proficiency is limited. This can make clients feel they are being treated like children.

Rate of Speech

Decrease your rate of speech and pause often. Many readers have had the experience of taking a foreign language class, then traveling to a country where that language is spoken and not understanding conversational speech because it was "too rapid." Similarly, many LCD clients benefit when clinicians use a slow speech rate. Clients also benefit when clinicians pause between sentences, because this gives the other party time to process what was just said.

Articulation in Connected Speech

Articulate each word clearly, but do not overexaggerate. Some clients relate that they do not understand because the "words run together so fast." For example, we usually coarticulate "How is it going?" as "Howzitgoing?" Clients do not know what "howzitgoing" is—it could be a type of food, a style of dress, or a particular kind of cloud formation. They do understand "How is it going?" when each word is produced separately and the copula is not contracted. This is especially true for clients raised in countries where British English is taught. Some Japanese and Koreans, for example, have difficulty with spoken U.S. English because it is not pronounced as precisely as the British English taught in Japanese and Korean schools.

Language Length and Complexity

Avoid the frequent use of long, polysyllabic words, as well as the use of slang, idiomatic speech, technical jargon, and abstract terminology. Use short sentences and phrases. It is very important not to use run-on, lengthy sentences. Clients have a hard time comprehending these.

Repeating Key Information

A thread running throughout this book is that clients need to hear key concepts several times. This is especially true for clients who speak English as a second, third, or fourth language. Repeating key concepts is important.

Nonverbal Cues and Body Language

Proxemics (the use of distance) and *kinesics* (the use of facial expressions and gestures) differ among cultures (Lane & Molyneaux, 1992). Be aware and accepting of nonverbal cues and body language that are culturally appropriate for particular clients. In many cultures, people are very sensitive to nuances of facial expression and body language. For example, among some members of the African American community, it is considered aggressive and disrespectful to make direct eye contact with an authority figure. Among some Latin Americans, kissing both cheeks in greeting is common (Tannen, 1994). Most Asian children are expected to listen and speak very little when interacting with adults (Hegde, 1995). Many Chinese individuals keep their faces expressionless, and Westerners may perceive Chinese as having poor eye contact (Cheng, 1991). Individuals from the Carolinian and Chamorro cultures tend to communicate extensively with their eyebrows. A speaker may raise the eyebrows to acknowledge a question, to greet another person, or to affirm or negate something that has been said (Hammer, 1994). Nonverbal cues are important, and it is helpful for clinicians to understand them and, as appropriate, to act in ways that are consistent with that family's culture.

Size of Interaction Groups

As noted in Chapter 1, there are two parties to an interview—the party that is conducting an interview and the party being interviewed. Encourage families to bring people who are important to them to a meeting. This can include friends, extended family members, and clergy. Many families will feel more comfortable and supported with these persons present.

However, do not overwhelm clients by bringing too many professionals into an interaction. In some interviewing and counseling situations, clients are surrounded by a coterie of professionals such as a speech-language pathologist, a surgeon, a psychologist, a physical therapist, an occupational therapist, and a nurse. This is intimidating to some clients. It is best to keep the number of professionals within a group as small as possible.

Flexibility

Be flexible and willing to provide assistance in establishing meetings. This could include meeting families in their homes, providing child care for siblings, or arranging transportation for families (Bondurant-Utz, 1994). Clinicians may need to meet with families in school cafeterias or on benches; at least one author (Kozloff, 1994) has met with parents in their cars. If clinicians insist on meeting with clients only in offices, they may not get to see certain clients or families at all.

Extra Time

Allow extra time for meetings and be patient. Meetings frequently take more time when clients do not speak English as a first language. It is important to avoid appearing hurried. Families from some backgrounds, such as the Native American culture, may not discuss their true concerns if they feel rushed (Anderson & Fenichel, 1989). Hispanic families may feel that if clinicians are in a hurry, they are showing the family disrespect or a lack of concern (Zuniga, 1992).

Suggestions for Using Interpreters

Professionals may need to utilize the services of interpreters during interviewing and counseling situations with clients who speak little or no English. Clinicians must be sure to use only those interpreters who have been trained properly; have good bilingual communication skills; act in professional manners; have the ability to relate well to members of their own cultural group; and understand and carry out their ethical responsibilities, including maintaining confidentiality.

Several reports in the literature give some excellent guidelines for situations where interpreters' services are utilized in meetings with clients and/or their families (Anderson, 1992; Culatta & Goldberg, 1995; Kayser, 1993; Langdon, 1992; Matsuda & O'Connor, 1993). These guidelines include the following:

• *Speak in short units and avoid professional jargon.* A major problem for many interpreters is that professionals speak in lengthy utterances that are technical and difficult to remember for translation.

• *Look at the client (or clients) as well as an interpreter when speaking and listening.* This is difficult for most clinicians to do—they tend to speak to and look at the interpreter only. This can make clients feel left out and unimportant. Clinicians must discipline themselves to make warm and caring eye contact with clients as they talk, and not just look at the interpreter.

• *Encourage the interpreter to translate clients' words without paraphrasing them as much as possible.* Some words or phrases have no direct translation, but clinicians need to hear exactly what clients say.

• *Explain the purpose, structure, and generally anticipated topics of discussion of an interviewing or counseling session to an interpreter beforehand.* Many interpreters report feeling "thrown into" various situations for which they are completely unprepared. While time is always at a premium, and clinicians do not usually have the luxury of long conversations with interpreters, clinicians should take some time to prepare interpreters for the situation ahead of them. Interpreters will be more effective if they are prepared, and they will be more successful in eliciting clients' cooperation when they can thoroughly explain rationales for clinicians' questions and requests. Interpreters must understand the interview questions completely and know how to record clients' responses (Roseberry-McKibbin, 1995).

• *Tape record the session,* if the family is comfortable with this. It is always helpful to have an audiotape to refer back to when questions arise.

• *Seat the interpreter as close to family members as possible.* Clients will be more comfortable if they are sitting near the interpreter.

• *Begin the meeting by introducing everyone and explaining the purpose of the meeting.* Clients should hear the names of each person in the meeting and understand what each person's role is. The purpose of the meeting may need to be reiterated several times throughout the meeting.

• *Be on hand at all times during the meeting.* Do not leave the room for coffee, for phone calls, or for errands. It is important to be present throughout in case questions or different areas of discussion arise.

• *Encourage family members to ask questions.* Many cultures consider it disrespectful to question professionals because they are viewed as authority figures. Clinicians need to ask interpreters to encourage family members to ask questions, if interpreters feel comfortable doing this and do not feel put on the spot.

• *Periodically check on the accuracy of translation and clients' understanding of what is being said.* Clinicians can ask family members to repeat instructions, but should avoid asking "Do you understand?" (Bondurant-Utz, 1994). Families may feel put on the spot and, to save face, say they do understand when in fact they do not. Having family members repeat what they have heard lets clinicians know whether or not the context of the interaction is being understood.

• *Discuss the session with the interpreter afterward.* This gives both individuals the opportunity to clarify information, ask questions, make comments, and discuss the meeting (Hegde & Davis, 1995).

• *Thank interpreters and pay them for their assistance.* Professionals need to treat interpreters with respect, dignity, and appreciation. Too often interpreters feel like they are spread very thin and are constantly rushing around, having their services utilized by professionals who may or may not appreciate the invaluable services provided. It behooves clinicians to remember that services to some families would be difficult if not impossible to provide without interpreters. In interviewing and counseling situations, which can be sensitive and highly charged, it is especially important to have available the services of competent interpreters who are well trained and who feel appreciated for the services they provide.

Suggestions for Increasing Personal Sensitivity

Many professionals truly desire to increase their sensitivity to and consequent effectiveness with clients from diverse backgrounds. The suggestions in the following sections, based in part on Lynch and Hanson (1992b) and Roseberry-McKibbin (1995), will assist individuals in upgrading their competence and knowledge to provide more effective services to LCD populations.

Use of Terminology

Do not use terms that have negative connotations. For example, terms, such as "at risk," "culturally deprived," and "culturally disadvantaged," imply that clients are being judged by an Anglo-European standard. This is ethnocentric and racist (Battle, 1993b).

Study of Cultures

Study the particular culture or cultures that are most common to your geographic area. As one frustrated student said to me several years ago, "There's no way I can learn about all these different cultures and remember everything about them!" This legitimate feeling is shared by many professionals, who feel overwhelmed as they face what can seem like a huge and endless task of learning details about different cultural groups. It is most efficacious to learn about the group or groups that clinicians will see most commonly in their particular geographic work area.

Names of Cultural Groups

Learn and use the names of cultural groups as assigned by the group members. This will save many misunderstandings (Battle, 1993b); however, each client and family must be taken on individual terms. For example, I had always used the term "Native American" when referring to members of that population. But, several years ago a native American student stated emphatically that she wished to be referred to as "American Indian." Another student, who was from Mexico, said she did not like the term "Latino." It is best to ascertain the preferences of each individual and family within a specific cultural group.

Common Words and Phrases

Learn and use some common words and greetings in the language(s) of the limited-English proficient families and clients served. Many professionals are monolingual English speakers. Clients generally appreciate a clinician's efforts to relate to them, even if it is only by using a few simple words or phrases in their language.

Interaction with Other Cultures

Interact, both during and outside of work, with members of the cultural communities being served. Professionals can take time to do simple things such as going to an ethnic grocery store, attending a church service conducted for a different cultural group, attending community cultural functions, going to centers for minority groups, and participating in various LCD holiday celebrations. Participating in these events provides opportunities to learn about other cultures in a broader manner than that provided by just seeing clients in one's office.

Utilizing Multicultural Contacts

Establish relationships with persons from the local LCD community who can serve as cultural informants and mediators. Such relationships are an invaluable part of working effectively with diverse clients and their families. Cultural mediators/informants/interpreters from clients' own backgrounds can frequently make more headway with certain individuals than professionals working alone. Some LCD clients feel more trust for and comfort with persons from their own communities.

Reading

Read what you can about the cultures and languages within the community. This information can be obtained from university and local libraries, as well as from individuals from various groups in the community. Several excellent sources of specific information about various cultural groups include Battle (1993a), Brigham Young University (1992), Cheng (1991), Lee and Richardson (1991), Lynch and Hanson (1992a), and Paniagua (1994).

Ethnographic Interviews

Ethnographic interviewing is used to gather information about a culture or individuals from that culture from a LCD informant's point of view (Cheng & Damico, 1994). Conduct ethnographic interviews with different members of the culture being served; do not interview just one member of that culture and base assumptions on that one person's viewpoints and perspectives. Questions can include, but should not be limited to, the following, which are based on and adapted from various authors (Bondurant-Utz, 1994; Cheng & Hammer, 1992; Lund & Duchan, 1993; and Mattes & Omark, 1991):

- What is the typical family size and constellation in this community?
- What is the typical family authority hierarchy?
- What are the roles of extended family members and siblings?
- What are the culture's parenting practices?
- What behaviors are expected for showing courtesy (e.g., avoiding eye contact with authority figures, not questioning professionals' decisions)?
- How does this cultural group view the role of special education? Of rehabilitation?
- How does the cultural group view the role of the impaired individual and the causes of handicapping conditions?
- What healing systems are used by group members? Would nonmedical or medical intervention violate beliefs in these systems?
- What role is played by factors such as poverty or immigrant/refugee status?
- What are the primary family or community concerns (e.g., health care, food, jobs)?
- What kind of community support is available for the family?
- What are the philosophical or religious influences on members of this culture?
- Do members of the culture perceive racism or discrimination from the mainstream culture? If so, how might this affect attitudes toward intervention?

Home Visits and Inquiring About Cultures

Visit families' homes if they are comfortable with this. Home visits, when appropriate, provide unique insight into individual families' ways of living and interacting. Ask clients to share important aspects of their culture with you. Many times professionals are afraid to ask clients about their cultural backgrounds. Although professionals must be careful not to pry or make clients uncomfortable, many clients are delighted to be asked to share information about their culture. Some of our best information about various LCD groups comes from asking clients to share about themselves and their culture!

Diversity within Cultures

Recognize the tremendous diversity that exists within each culture. Learning about other cultures is an exciting, dynamic, and ongoing process. Clinicians can never assume that because they have read a chapter in a book about "Asians," or attended one or two workshops about "Hispanics," that they can settle comfortably into, or operate effectively, from that small knowledge base, as though all Asian or Hispanic clients possess the characteristics learned from those sources. Students and professionals must constantly respect and be aware of the great diversity that exists within each culture (Taylor & Clarke, 1994), and not stereotype individuals or try to put them into rigid, preexisting frameworks into which they may or may not fit. Each client and each family is unique!

Diversity with Languages

Recognize the diversity within various languages. For example, people can go to any part of the United States or Canada and understand the English used. However, in many other countries, there is a great variety of languages and dialects within the individual country. For example, I was raised on the small island of Tablas in the Philippines. Residents of Odiongan spoke Odionganon as the local vernacular. On the other side of Tablas, in the town of Looc, residents spoke Loocnon. Both were distinctively different languages.

More than 1,200 indigenous languages are spoken in the Pacific Islands (Campbell, 1989), and many of these languages are mutually unintelligible. There are more than 87 dialects in China (Cheng, 1991). As previously mentioned, clinicians must be aware that people from the same general language group may speak mutually unintelligible dialects of a given language. When clinicians use interpreters, they need to make sure the interpreter and client have at least one dialect in common so that they can understand each other.

Religious Influence

The influence of religion and religious beliefs was addressed in Chapter 3. Be sensitive to the role that religion plays in clients' lives. Religions impact on services to and interactions with clients. For example, during the month of Ramadan, most Muslims do not have food or drink between sunrise and sundown; thus, clinicians might not want to offer food or drink to Muslim clients during Ramadan. Buddhists have a special three-day holiday in August (Nellum-Davis, 1993); therefore, Buddhist families may not be available for sessions during these days. It also may be difficult for some Buddhist families to accept certain forms of medical intervention, such as cleft palate surgery, because they believe that disabled children will be reincarnated to a whole form (Anderson & Fenichel, 1989). There are many other possible influences of religion and religious beliefs.

Sharing Information

As clinicians learn about LCD clients and their backgrounds, the information should be shared with others. This is helpful for everyone because personal and professional experiences benefit other clinicians and the clients they serve (Hegde & Davis, 1995).

Concluding Comments

As we move into the twenty-first century, exciting challenges await our profession. One of these major challenges is to effectively serve an increasingly LCD population whose members have unique characteristics, needs, and expectations. There are a number of areas clinicians need to consider when working with LCD clients and families. Many different areas to consider are addressed in this chapter. Learning about other cultures, languages, and values of clients for ourselves is a continual journey—always interesting, sometimes challenging, and most of all, deeply rewarding. Our diverse clients always serve as a reminder of one of life's great truths—we must never stop growing and learning to live well together.

Chapter *9*

Working with Difficult Situations

In a helping profession such as ours, most of a clinician's work is with people—patients, family members, or other caregivers—who are concerned about the problems being experienced and are eager to assist. These people are typically cooperative and often appreciative of a clinician's efforts. Working with this vast majority of clients and their families is a true source of personal pleasure and professional gratification. There are, however, some situations that are not as pleasant, at least initially, and some individuals are simply less cooperative than others.

This chapter addresses certain situations and events in interviewing and counseling sessions that are sometimes confusing or frustrating to some clinicians. However, it is important to note that, like beauty, "difficulty" or what is perceived as being a "difficult situation" is often in the eyes of the beholder. What is perceived as being a very difficult situation for one person may not be for someone else. This often relates to an individual's level of knowledge of self and others, experience, and probably most important, a clinician's outlook and approaches to people and clinical work. It is important to realize that there is no magical formula for working with the more difficult situations or even people. Rather, clinical workers need to react (or not react) to situations at hand, and develop steps for working with different circumstances on a case-by-case basis. There are, however, some basic principles that help clinicians understand what is happening and, often, react appropriately in more difficult situations. Several general, introductory suggestions include the following:

- Make yourself stay calm while minimizing your own levels of emotional involvement. Stay cool and in control.
- Try to understand as fully as possible what might be motivating or happening with the other party.
- Identify the specific behaviors, attitudes, or other factors that are of concern to you.
- Do not allow yourself to overreact negatively to anything that is said—at least not visually. Your heart may be pounding and stomach churning, but do not let the other person see this.
- When dealing with individuals who are culturally or linguistically different, and certain values or attitudes are demonstrated, try to understand the other party's viewpoint or actions in a cultural perspective.

The application of these suggestions should be reconsidered while reading this chapter. It is also worth remembering that, in Moses' (1985) words, clinicians typically deal with "crazy making circumstances, not crazy people" (p. 84). People with communicative disorders sometimes come into clinical settings frustrated, bewildered, confused, depressed, angry, and/or filled with fears about what today and the future will bring. Clients and their caregivers may be cooperative, concerned, and caring—or, they may be what clinicians perceive as uncooperative, apathetic, or having counterproductive attitudes and behaviors. Dealing with a communicative difficulty can indeed be a "crazy making circumstance" for clients, families, friends, and others. The clinician's task is to help these people deal effectively and productively with such circumstances.

Potentially Difficult Communication Behaviors

There are several types of behaviors that, while they may not occur every day, are seen in some clinical settings. These include resistance, denial, questioning, discrepancies, shifts of conversational focus, "recurrent themes," and gaps of information. Some of these—certain types of resistance, denial, and some forms of questioning—are similar to or are even related to active defense mechanisms, which were discussed in Chapter 3. Other aspects of client behavior—discrepancies, conversational shifts, recurrent references, and information gaps—have more to do with the flow of conversation and information between a clinician and a client. These aspects of client behavior may result from a defensive reaction, a lapse of memory, or are just inadvertent. Thus, clinicians try to assess why they are occurring and work with these areas. Of course, sometimes clinicians are fully successful doing this; other times they are less successful than desired. A good deal of a clinician's success in this area begins by identifying what is really happening.

Resistance

Resistance is a natural phenomenon that occurs to some degree in many, if not most relationships. Resistance usually occurs when individuals fear change or are uncertain about some situation (Okun, 1992; Orr & Adams, 1987). In a clinical setting, resistance can be expressed by behaviors such as tardiness, an abrupt changing of topic, "forgetfulness," subtle or overt forms of inattention, silence, disagreement with something shared, or the failure to follow through on suggestions (the hearing aid not worn, the homework assignments not practiced, the appointment with the physician not made, and so on).

Resistance tends to occur more frequently early in a clinical relationship such as surrounding assessment activities or early in the treatment process. Brammer (1993) lists several of what he calls the "realities" of a new relationship, each of which can result in resistance:

- *It is not easy to receive help.*
- *It is difficult to commit oneself to change.*
- *It is difficult to submit to the influence of a helper; help is a threat to esteem, integrity, and independence.*
- *It is not easy to trust strangers and to be open with them.*
- *It is not easy to see one's problems clearly at first.*
- *Sometimes problems seem too large, too overwhelming, or too unique to share them easily.*
- *Some cultural traditions deprecate giving and receiving help outside the family.* (p. 56)

Resistance also occurs when there is disagreement about something said or done, or when something has been misunderstood. The patient who disagrees with a clinician's comments or recommendations is likely to resist, in one way or another, the clinician's findings, conclusions, or suggestions. Also, patients who develop ill feelings toward a clinician tend to be resistant. The ill feelings may be a reaction to a clinician's attitude, something said, a gesture, or another form of body language. It is important for clinicians to evaluate whether they are doing something that is engendering resistance, or whether the resistance has other causes. For example, if a parent does not really believe a child needs treatment, but allows the youngster to be enrolled for services anyway, ambivalence or resistance may occur. The parent might not even be conscious of such feelings. In such a case, clinicians try to overcome the ambivalence or resistance by working with the parent's feelings about the need for services—the feelings that are the source of the problem.

Another source of resistance is change itself (Brammer, 1993). Consider the following explanation, from MacLean and Gould (1988), of how change and risk apply to the experience of resistance.

> *Change implies the giving up of something old, and learning, doing, being something new. There is a sense in which the old has to be unlearned, and new ways relearned. It is not surprising that clients (and all of us) tend to stick with what is known—the habitual, familiar way of behaving. Giving up these old ways [is] like giving up familiar friends, there are risks involved.* (p. 33)

Often a client's resistance can be overcome in time, as the two parties accumulate experiences together and trust and faith grow. Lavorato and McFarlane (1988) describe resistance and one approach used in the beginning with a voice case:

> *For some individuals, whether to engage in voice therapy or not is a major decision. Perhaps they do not understand the reason for it, or do not want to change their voice, or spend the time and money required, or just feel silly engaging in therapy. Advising and explaining the rationale for therapy is sufficient for most clients. Playing audiotapes or videotapes of previous successes can be an inducement for others. The case that follows required a different approach. The client was a nurse who was "sprawled out" in the waiting room and stood reluctantly, looking angry, when greeted.*
>
> CLINICIAN: *And what is your concern about your speech?*
>
> CLIENT: *I have none. I just went to the doctor with an ear problem, that's all. There's nothing wrong with my throat.*
>
> CLINICIAN: *What did he say was wrong with your throat?*
>
> CLIENT: *He said my vocal cords look irritated and that I was talking wrong. Hell, I know how I talk! I've been husky all my life. So is the rest of my family. We all talk like this. We talk loudly, and all the women have deep voices. He has followed me for my ear problem for two weeks, and all he talks about is my throat. I don't have the time or interest to work on my voice.*
>
> CLINICIAN: *That's kind of irritating. You don't need another problem in your life.*
>
> CLIENT: *You'd better believe it. I'm divorced and have complete responsibility for my children. I'm busy.*
>
> CLINICIAN: *Look. I'm concerned about your not wanting to be here. I respect your feelings about this and feel that you should not be forced into anything. At this point, what would you like me to do? If you want me to cancel this session, I will do it right now.*
>
> CLIENT: (Less abrupt, more receptive in posture, tone of voice, choice of words, rate of speech.) *Well, what will happen if I don't follow through with his recommendation to see you?*

CLINICIAN: (Explains the possible outcomes of her problem if left untreated.)

CLIENT: *I do talk a lot. I lecture—and wish that I didn't have to do that. A lot of times, my voice is almost gone by the time I finish a lecture. I don't really like my voice—it distracts from my message.*

CLINICIAN: *Some of my clients say they begin to get nervous when the voice begins to go and they have more talking to do.*

CLIENT: *It is very distracting. Not only that, but my throat occasionally gets an irritated feeling, and it is uncomfortable talking.*

CLINICIAN: *I know what you mean.*

CLIENT: *What is involved in voice therapy? How many times would I have to come in?*

The client agreed to an evaluation and to initiate therapy. Giving her the option to do so was critical. It put her back in control and indicated the clinician's respect for her feelings and situation. It also led her to be more open about her problem. (pp. 246-247)

Rejection—the conscious, active unwillingness to agree with the clinician's descriptions, interpretations, conclusions, or recommendations—is a more emphatic form of resistance. When rejection occurs, clinicians need to carefully consider a client's underlying feelings. This can be done by pleasantly but directly reflecting a client's messages.

"You feel differently about it. Tell me about how you are feeling about _____."

"You don't fully agree with that, do you?"

"Tell me about your concerns with this recommendation."

Sometimes clinicians need to use a more direct comment to get at the source of the rejection.

"You are very quiet today. Tell me about it."

"You seem uncomfortable talking about _____."

"I sense that you would rather talk about _____ than _____ today."

"This is the third time you've been late this week. This seems to be a pattern. I'd like to know what's really bothering you."

Resistance from some clients from diverse backgrounds may occur for several reasons, including trust issues. Certain cultures are also less direct than the mainstream culture, so a highly direct clinician can engender resistance when working with someone from such a background. Resistance may relate to how a culture views communicative problems, or how problems are dealt with. In some Native American tribes, the extended family is responsible for taking care of problems—outside intervention is less acceptable. Many devout Muslims believe that only Allah knows the future, so planning more than a few weeks ahead does not make much sense. Discussing long-term plans and strategies may not seem as important to these individuals as clinicians would like (Nellum-Davis, 1993). Therefore what might appear as resistance is reflective of cultural outlook and beliefs.

Denial

Denial is a response that clinicians see with some frequency with communicative disorders. For example, audiologists often see patients whose hearing has been impaired for long periods of time. As a frustrated spouse might complain,

> "I've told him for years to go get his hearing tested. But oh no, not him and his pride! He always said his hearing was as sharp as a tack. Trouble is he couldn't hear me tell him he was wrong."

Some parents deny, sometimes for long periods of time, that their child actually has a speech, language, or hearing problem. A number of clinicians have been told on more than one occasion that "I am not concerned about it; he'll outgrow it," or "He'll start talking. His father didn't talk until he was four years old!" Failure to recognize a problem and the use of rationalization are forms of denial. *Denial* is a defense mechanism people employ when they are not ready to admit that a problem exists and begin remedying the situation. This is sometimes seen in patients who are "just not ready" (see Brammer, Abrego, & Shostrom, 1993). Like resistance, it is a response that people may not be conscious of using.

Denial is a very common characteristic, for example, of chemically dependent persons and their families. The chemically dependent person, the family, friends, coworkers, superiors—sometimes no one is ready to fully acknowledge the problem, its ramifications, or its solutions. A form of denial is *minimizing,* making some problem out to be less than it actually is. Again, in the field of chemical dependence, minimization is encountered frequently. For example, when asking a practicing alcoholic or drug addict the quantity of alcohol or drugs being used, it is common for respondents to report a figure that is considerably less than what is really being used. The same person may also vehemently convey that the drinking or using has little affect on self, family, friends, school, or job. This person is minimizing the problem and its effects.

Patients and families who are denying the existence of something or minimizing a problem and its consequences need time, knowledge, and support to help them acknowledge and cope with what is actually happening and begin to accept what needs to be done. This process sometimes takes time—it certainly takes the understanding, the support, and often the caring and persistent direct assistance of a clinician.

For some individuals, denial is a temporary solution along the road to understanding and agreement. It acts to help them "buy time" while evaluating if what they feel is true—and what is in their best interests or in the best interests of the family member with a communicative disorder. Clinicians need to realize that even if clients or loved ones are denying something outwardly, they may still—behind the cover of the denial—be contemplating whether the information is true and the clinician's feelings or descriptions are accurate. Thus, many clinicians have heard comments like the following:

> "When you first told me my son would not improve without therapy, I really didn't believe it. But the more we thought about how he's doing and what you told us, the more we began to think you were right."

> "I know I said I can hear fine and don't need a hearing aid. But I've been noticing that it is sometimes a little hard to hear everything. Can we talk about it again? I'm still not going to get a hearing aid, but I want to talk about it and make sure I understand what you said."

These examples illustrate how a patient who denied something has thought about the information conveyed and altered a stance of complete denial that was originally taken.

In some cases, clinicians need to very candid with someone who is denying the existence of a problem; for example:

> "I have worked intensively with your father for a month now and he's made very little progress. All of the medical reports indicate that he has severe brain damage. The brain is just not working like it once did. But you still seem to feel that he will be fine again in time. I know you would like to see major improvement, but it seems like it's difficult for you to come to grips with the fact that he is not going to be the same as he was before . . ."

> "I know you have felt that Jason was going to start speaking at any time. But he's almost four now, and he's still not talking. I'm feeling like we may have two problems. One is Jason's inability to talk. The other is that you are having a hard time dealing with this problem. I think this is difficult for you to accept. Let's talk about how you are feeling."

Neither of these examples is necessarily typical of most clinical discussions with patients or family members. However, the examples do illustrate the types of conversations clinicians need to conduct in certain situations of denial.

Such degrees of candor, however, are not appropriate with some clients from linguistically or culturally diverse backgrounds, particularly those from cultures placing a greater value on indirectness. It is also important to consider whether an individual from a different background is truly denying a problem in the traditional Anglo-European sense—it is possible that a particular difficulty is not necessarily viewed as being a problem within this group, or that the notion of intervention is inconsistent with cultural or even religious values. Taylor and Clarke

(1994) remark that "societies seem to have different perceptions of what aspects of communication, if any, they consider pathologic and what to do about it, if anything" (p. 109).

There are instances in which identifying someone as disabled or impaired stigmatizes the individual. In the Philippines or China, for example, the idea of "deformity" may be viewed as being a curse so an individual is ostracized from society. In other cultures, it is particularly difficult for some fathers to accept that there may be anything wrong with their sons. Such views can be seen as denial or resistance, but they also reflect cultural values.

Questioning

There can be many reasons why some clients question a clinician's assessment conclusions or treatment suggestions. For one thing, a clinician might be wrong. For example, a clinician told one patient's parents that her child would outgrow her articulation problems. Unfortunately, an oral examination had not been performed adequately; the presence of a severe ankyloglossia (tongue-tie) was undetected. This child could not have outgrown the speech problem nor would therapy have remedied the speech difficulties; rather, surgical intervention was needed. Fortunately the parents had questioned the earlier diagnosis and sought a second opinion.

Some clients may also question a clinician's diagnosis or prognosis because they are simply unable, at that point, to fully accept what the clinician has found. This really is not an uncommon reaction to many events in life. As indicated previously, denying a diagnosis provides a temporary solution to the inability to understand and cope with what is happening. Likewise, questioning a diagnosis or asking for a second opinion should not necessarily be interpreted as an attack on the professional. Rather, it may be an important step toward understanding and acknowledgment (Cunningham & Davis, 1985).

Sometimes clinicians see patients and families who do not ask questions; for example, the passive nonlisteners described in Chapter 2 (see "Listening and Activity Levels"). Also, individuals from some cultures (e.g., Hispanic or Japanese) tend not to openly disagree or question clinicians in areas of disagreement or confusion out of respect for that person.

As with resistance and denial, then, it is important to realize that there are many possible sources for questioning behavior—or the lack of questioning. Resistance, denial, and questioning a clinician can all act as hesitations, as interruptions of the diagnostic or therapeutic process. They can be engendered by the clinician, or they can have causes independent of the professional services provided. In any case, clinicians are obligated to help clients understand the situation as well as possible. This is most easily accomplished by providing accurate information, genuine support, and appropriate summaries of findings and conclusions.

Discrepancies

Ivey (1994) describes several types of discrepancies and mixed messages that can occur in clinical situations.

• *Discrepancy between nonverbal behaviors.* The individual displays a pleasant, "no problem" type of smile accompanied by a tightly clenched fist.

• *Discrepancy between two or more statements.* "My son is perfect, but he just doesn't respect me." "I understand what you are saying but still think an in-the-ear aid would be better."

• *Discrepancy between what one says and what one does.* Individuals say they are "behind you 100%" and promise to do everything possible to help, but consistently fail to complete the homework requested.

• *Discrepancy between a statement and nonverbal behavior.* The client verbally relates that the stuttering does not bother him; meanwhile tears swell in his eyes and the fists are tightly clenched.

• *Discrepancy between the views of different people.* A father and mother disagree about the impact of a communicative disorder on their child. Brother and sister tell conflicting versions of how much their father's hearing is affecting their everyday lives. (Adapted from Ivey, 1994, pp. 78-80.)

Often clinicians can clear up a discrepancy or mixed message by probing into the area of question. This probe is usually sufficient to resolve accidental or inadvertent discrepancies. For example, suppose a client indicated at one point that the hearing seemed better in the right ear, but later said the hearing was better in the left ear. Rather unobtrusively, a clinician could say something like, "Let me make sure I have it straight. Tell me again which one is your better ear." The patient's response could then be summarized back to the client for reconfirmation; for example, "So it is the hearing in your left ear that does not seem as good." The clinician may want to probe this again at a later time for further confirmation that the left ear is of primary concern.

At other times, clinicians need to explicitly identify a discrepancy for the patient as in the following examples:

"Mr. Smith, you mentioned that Johnny started talking at about two years of age. Mrs. Smith, you seem to recall that it may have been as late as age four. Let's talk about this . . ."

"Sandy, you said your stuttering is not really a problem and that it doesn't really bother you. But it looked like you were about to cry when you said that. Tell me how you're feeling about your stuttering."

"Robert, you say you like your hearing aid and that it helps you hear better. But your teacher says you are not wearing it in class. I'm confused. You say you like it and it helps, but you aren't using it. Can you help me make sense of this?"

Most discrepancies and mixed messages can be resolved, or at least understood better, with such confronting techniques. An even more direct form of confrontation is reserved for extreme cases.

> "On one hand, you are telling me how concerned you are about Tom and his problems, and that you will help in any way possible. On the other hand, his home practice is not getting done. What you are saying does not seem to mesh with what is actually happening. Help me with this inconsistency."

> "You say that your stuttering is no big deal and it doesn't really bother you. But you almost cry every time I ask you about it. It seems like you are really hurting. Your words are saying 'no big deal,' but everything else is saying that it is a big deal. Tell me about these inconsistencies."

Certain disorders can also present a form of discrepancy. For example, many aphasics exhibit "yes/no" confusions in their speech—"yes" sometimes means "no," or vice versa, or the two terms are used inconsistently. Clinicians need to be sensitive when working with some members of linguistically and culturally different populations. Certainly a language barrier can cause confusing or seemingly discrepant responses. Clinicians sometimes are also frustrated by perceived discrepancies between what someone agrees to do, and the lack of follow-up that occurs. As Chan (1992a) notes:

> *While apparently concurring in some manner (through failure to express or defend an alternative point of view) or ostensibly indicating agreement, Filipinos may actually be privately opposed to the issue at hand. Thus . . . mistakes will go unmentioned, questions unasked, and issues unsettled.* (p. 288)

Out of respect, some parents from the Hispanic culture also may not openly disagree with clinicians; thus, they may give the appearance of following certain directions or agreeing to something without fully intending to follow-up (Langdon, 1992). Discrepancies also occur among family members, particularly when some within the family acknowledge a difficulty but others (often fathers) do not.

Conversational Shifts

A shift in the conversation may mean that a given subject has been discussed fully and that it is now time to move on. A conversational shift that is distinctly abrupt, however, can indicate that interviewees or counselees are feeling that they are revealing too much about themselves (or their parents, children, or significant other). An abrupt shift in conversation is also an indication that some topic is too painful or too sensitive to discuss (Shertzer & Stone, 1980). Thus, abrupt conversational shifts can be unstated comments that "I do not want to discuss that," "I am not ready to talk about that now," or "That's none of your business."

During a first meeting, it is sometimes best not to force an issue that is so sensitive to a patient; rather, it may be better to wait until a more secure and trusting relationship is developed. Clinicians should make a mental note of the conversational shift at this point; actually stopping to write a note about it tends to engender suspicion, distrust, or fear. Sometimes it is helpful to return briefly to the topic at least once more during a session. If the same reaction (that is, another abrupt conversational shift) occurs, clinicians can be pretty sure the topic is a sensitive one. If needed, this topic can be pursued more directly at a later time.

The mother of one of my clients provided a good example of an abrupt conversational shift away from a sensitive area. During the first meeting, I asked her when she first noticed her son's speech problem. She quickly changed the topic with the question, "Can you help my son or not?" I gently moved back into the sensitive area twice more later during the first session, and each time she abruptly changed the subject. It was obvious that, for whatever reason, she felt very sensitive about the question.

The child was subsequently enrolled for therapy and our relationship as professional and parent developed well. After the child's third therapy session, I asked the mother to join me in my office for a brief chat. We talked briefly about the progress we had seen to that point. Then I commented:

> "The first time we met, I asked you about when you first noticed your son's speech problem. This was not an area you were ready to discuss at that time. If you are still not ready to talk about it, that's OK. If it is an area of importance to either you or your son, please feel free to talk about it. Either way is OK."

The mother thought about my comments for a couple of moments, then shared the following:

> "I knew immediately that you knew there was a problem, but thank you for not pushing me. I just couldn't talk about it then! Kevin [her husband], my mother, Kevin's parents, and my sisters all said Darrell had a speech problem and that I needed to get it taken care of. I guess I just couldn't face Darrell being anything but normal. Now I know I was wrong. I've really messed him up by waiting so long. He'll never catch up, will he? It's all my fault for being so stupid!"

It was important for her to express what was really bothering her. This provided us with an opportunity to deal with her guilt, to look again at the prognosis for her son, and to establish an even more positive and trusting relationship. As she and her son left that day, her final comments were:

"Thank you again for not pushing me when I couldn't have told you, and thank you for asking me again when I could. I needed to tell someone who could understand. Thank you again."

Conversational shifts can occur at any time during diagnostic or treatment sequences. The point that needs to be emphasized is that conversational shifts are often meaningful and important. Clinicians need to develop the habit of mentally tucking away sensitive topics that are revealed by conversational shifts. Such shifts need to be addressed at some point, but it is often unproductive to pursue or confront them too early during a relationship.

Recurrent Themes

Clinicians sometimes find an interviewee returning several times to one or more particular topics of discussion (Shertzer & Stone, 1980). For example, a patient may return to the subject of the costs of services, to the cause of a problem, or to a prognosis. There is no limit to the number of recurrent themes possible. Recurrent themes represent areas of particular concern to interviewees. At some point, clinicians need to address these themes or topics. The themes will recur until a client's concerns have been resolved, or—even worse—the client stops mentioning them altogether out of the belief that the clinician is not listening, is unconcerned or uncaring, or is incapable of helping. Thus, a clinician's failure to respond can lead to having two problems to deal with. The first problem is the area addressed by the recurrent theme; the second is negative feelings about not "picking up on" the area of concern.

There is another reason for clinicians to deal directly with recurrent themes. When clients and their concerns are not yet resolved, it is not possible for them to concentrate fully on other areas of importance. For example, if patients are preoccupied with the costs of services, they will have difficulty staying focused on a clinician's diagnosis, treatment recommendations, or other areas of discussion.

The content of recurrent themes dictates how clinicians deal with them. When the focuses of recurrent themes are on past actions or events, these may need to be discussed as springboards to the present and the future. Deep-seated feelings of guilt may need to be discussed openly, or clinicians may need to make a referral for appropriate counseling.

The type of cognitive or behavioral counseling discussed in Chapter 7 is helpful with many clients. Clinicians provide a new cognitive set; reinforce thoughts and verbalizations that are productive and appropriate; and punish or do not reinforce tangential, less important, or unproductive recurrent themes that have already been addressed.

Information Gaps

Gaps in information occur for a number of reasons. For example, a military parent may have been away from home for protracted periods of time; some adoptive parents (particularly children adopted overseas or from some drug- or alcohol-dependent birth mothers) do not have information about their child's prenatal, birth, or early developmental history; or a patient may have been comatose or under heavy medication and have little, if any, recall of certain events or time periods. There are other factors that influence the recall of information.

Time. Ask the parent of a two-year-old when her child started walking and you will probably get a precise answer. Ask the same mother the identical question 15 years later and the answer is often more general or tentative. This reflects the amount of time that has occurred since some event in question.

"Pecking order." Ask a parent when his first child started to talk and you will usually get a pretty quick, reliable answer. Ask the same parent when the fourth of his six children started to talk and see what happens. You may hear something like, "Well, let me think about that for a moment. Lisa came after Terry. John wasn't born yet, so…." In general, it is more difficult for many parents to recall certain specifics about each child when there is a larger number of children.

Simultaneously occurring factors. Ask a parent of a three-year-old who was not employed outside the home when her child first developed two-word phrases. Now ask another parent of a three-year-old the same question, but assume that this second parent was involved in a career and involved with ongoing care of a terminally ill parent at the same time. You can guess which parent is more likely to know the answer to the question.

The effects of multiple, simultaneously occurring factors is seen with many recent immigrants and their families. Some refugee families have lived in several countries, in different places within these countries, and experienced a number of simultaneously occurring hardships during this time (bureaucracy, unfamiliar customs, health issues, within-family separations).

Memory, health, environmental, and other factors. Memory, health, environment, focus of attention, and a plethora of other factors all affect what is remembered. An individual's personality and intellectual differences are also significant factors. For example, some two-year-olds are almost nonverbal and others can put together semantically, syntactically, and morphologically correct sentences. Some 20-year-olds do not know how to use a dictionary (or even spell it) while others can fully explain nuclear fission or how television works. There are elderly people who cannot remember what they ate at a just-completed meal and others who can recall and marshal incredibly complex details from their past. There are many factors that can create knowledge gaps. Clinicians need to carefully interpret why an information gap is occurring before overinferring anything from it.

Other types of gaps. Having said there are many reasons for information gaps, there is another potential sources of such gaps. For example, as Shertzer and Stone (1980) comment:

> *Gaps, particularly if they are repeated, may be significant to understanding the client. A counselee who describes the members of his or her family but omits mentioning a brother or sister leaves a gap that may have meaning fundamental to understanding the problem.* (p. 299)

Clinicians working with communicative disorders sometimes find similar gaps in the presentation of information related to family interactions, to the identification of a problem, or to someone's attempts to work with the problem. When such information gaps occur, clinicians may need to further explore these areas.

Emotions, Attitudes, and Behaviors

Anger

Anger is often a reaction to feeling frustrated, afraid, or threatened (Cormier & Hackney, 1987). Anger is also a common reaction to feelings of discomfort, desperation, or powerlessness—for example, when everyday situations get out of control. A long line at the supermarket, poor service in a restaurant, a poor grade on a paper, a missed deadline, a rejection, accidental breakage of a valued possession—these are examples of everyday situations that potentially provoke anger.

Different people have different ways of showing or dealing with anger. People with "short fuses" become quickly and demonstrably angry and may openly express their hostility. Other people, meanwhile, may become angry but consciously endeavor not to show their anger. Still others, "taking things in stride," seem to handle provocative situations passively, without apparent emotion. Such an individual may not even consciously experience anger in such situations. Imagine an overcrowded waiting room of a busy physician who is running several hours behind schedule. The room is filled with agitated people, all reacting differently to the situation. Some patients read quietly, others pace, some check their watches every few minutes, others ask the receptionist how much longer it will be, others ask to use the phone, and still others complain bitterly to unknown strangers about the delay. The point is, people experience and exhibit frustration and anger in different ways.

Illness certainly tends to engender anger (Enelow & Swisher, 1986). The level of discomfort patients feel—as well as their fears for their health, their recovery, and their finances, or their frustration dealing with bureaucratic procedures, poor interagency cooperation, or uncooperative insurance companies—are all factors that may influence the degree and frequency of anger clinicians see, irrespective of the type of setting in which they work.

Clinicians themselves can be a source for angry feelings—when they are perceived as being brusque, sarcastic, condescending, uncaring, or even thoughtless (McFarlane, Fujiki, & Brinton, 1984). Thus, when evaluating the reasons for a patient's anger, professionals should always examine their own behavior to see if they are responsible for provoking the responses. Of course there are other times when a patient's anger has been generated elsewhere, and the clinician just happens to be the first person available for its ventilation. Consider, for example, the unfortunate clinician who is the first person to see a now-irate client who was running late and then had to drive around 45 minutes searching for a parking place. You know who is going to hear about it!

There are also some individuals whose whole lives seem surrounded by anger. As Enelow and Swisher (1986) write:

> *The chronically angry man or woman is always a difficult problem for the interviewer. Often his difficulties are related to anger. The clinician must keep in mind that he is not the primary or sole target of this anger. Observation and the history of the patient should make clear that this is part of the patient's life style.* (p. 97)

Although it is a possibility to be pondered, usually it is not the case that the clinician has engendered the client's anger. Stroke patients who have been rendered unable to communicate typically are not angry with the clinician. Rather, these patients may be angry and frustrated about what has occurred, the excruciating fears associated with newly encountered problems (Am I going to die? Will I ever be able to speak again? Or, to understand others?), the horribly scary fears for the future (Am I always going to be like this? What will my spouse or children do? How can I afford this? Can I ever go back to work?), or even difficulties performing the tasks presented by the clinician.

Clinicians who work with acquired neurologic disorders, such as aphasia, often ask patients to identify, name, or describe the functions of common objects (a ball, pen, stamp). These are tasks that would be asked of a one- or two-year old child under normal communicative circumstances. Such task presentations are needed to evaluate current levels of communicative functioning. But such tasks can certainly be perceived as very demeaning and serve to highlight the communicative difficulties being experienced, leading to feelings of frustration and anger.

When dealing with this type of anger, clinicians should realize that it is probably not them as a person who is creating the irritation. When treating such patients, it is helpful to be warm, supportive, and understanding. One 22-year-old patient who was a very talented professional musician had been in a near-fatal automobile accident. At the time he was first seen, the patient seemed to comprehend everything rather well but was barely able to phonate an "ah" on command. About halfway through the evaluative session, he had a violent temper tantrum (which is rather common among patients with injuries to the brain). Test items went flying through the air and he screamed an "ah" that seemed to exceed 110 or 120 decibels. When the tantrum subsided (tantrums do subside if you wait long enough), I quietly asked, "Were you mad at me, mad at what I was asking you to do, or mad at what has happened to you?" He responded by pointing to himself and forced out a vowelized approximation of the word "me." This provided an excellent opportunity for me to acknowledge that he had gone through a horrible experience and express the desire to help him learn to communicate again. After this, and again only in forced and labored vowels, he said "thank you" and reached out to touch my hand. We held hands for a few moments, then it was back to work with one very motivated, cooperative patient.

As I reflect on my encounter with this severely injured young person, any other type of response from me would have been less productive for him. Responding with anger, trying to settle him down during the tantrum, telling him that such outbursts occur commonly with brain injuries, moralizing that 22-year-olds should not behave like that, or responding in any other way simply would not have been in his best interests. No other response would have created the warm, cooperative relationship that subsequently emerged during that session and the sessions that followed.

Overprotection

The instinct to protect is basic for all animals, including humans. We protect ourselves, our family and friends, and our possessions in order to prevent loss or harm and to ensure survival. We use seat belts to prevent severe injury in the event of an accident, take vitamins to maintain health and avoid illness, lock doors to prevent uninvited intrusions, and so forth. Protection is a basic human need.

Problems emerge, however, when people try to overprotect those for whom they care. An overprotected individual is shielded from opportunities to experience life, to become more independent, to make optimal progress. Overprotection often creates a variety of strains and imbalances with basic family structures (Cunningham & Davis, 1985). A spouse, a parent, a child, a teacher—anyone with deep feelings of love or concern for another person can be overly protective. It is not unusual to encounter overprotective attitudes in one whose spouse is experiencing a severe communicative disorder (aphasia, for example) or in the parents of a child exhibiting a severe speech, language, or hearing difficulty. Of course, parents can be overprotective of normally developing children as well as those who have some kind of impairment.

The notion of being overprotective is culturally relative. Mainstream society values freedom and independence; some other cultures place less importance on these values. Some Pacific Island families, for example, protect physically impaired children and do not expect them to become independent (Fitzgerald & Barker, 1993). In the Micronesian Chamorro and Carolinian cultures, many parents acquiesce to their children's desires to minimize the frustration of those who have had medical problems and illnesses (Hammer, 1994).

Arambula (1992) notes that some Hispanic families may feel

> *that the elderly family member (e.g., stroke victim) has "had a difficult life" and that it is the family's turn to take care of the patient. The philosophy of "helping patients help themselves" on which rehabilitation specialists base their effort to instill a sense of independence in the patient often conflicts with what the Hispanic patient and family desire.* (p. 385)

Clearly there are cultural interpretations to what is deemed taking care of responsibilities, appropriate levels of protection, and overprotection. However, excessive overprotection that interferes with appropriate progress may need to be dealt with clinically in a number of cases. Typically, the least effective method of dealing with overprotection initially is confrontation. Even alluding to overprotectiveness often engenders the type of defensiveness that underpins the overprotection in the first place.

Frequently, a more effective method to use in dealing with overprotection is to engage the person who is overprotecting in helping devise strategies and methods to help develop more independent functioning for the person being overprotected. Clinicians seek the overprotective person's help in encouraging more independence and self-reliance on the part of the patient. A clinician's chances for success are much greater with the help of the overprotective person—whether that person is ever apprised of the overprotectiveness. This allows the person who is overprotecting to continue to be somewhat "overprotective" while helping devise and implement methods that will increase the patient's overall independence—but the result is reduced overprotectiveness.

Entitlement

All patients are entitled to appropriate, effective, caring services. There are a number of factors that relate to people's feelings of what they are entitled to, and these feelings or expectations can influence clinicians' views toward their clients. The area of time and patients' expectations of what a professional–client relationship should be are important considerations. As Reyes (1994) comments:

> *Many Western cultures place much emphasis and importance on adherence to structured schedules, whereas other cultures may view time as a relative concept, with the quality of interpersonal relationships taking priority over schedules and punctuality. . . . People who are event-oriented tend to be more concerned that an activity be completed, regardless of the length of time required, and emphasize unscheduled participation rather than carefully structured activities.* (p. 165)

Clinicians do meet what has been called the "entitled client" from time to time (Edinburg, Zinberg, & Kelman, 1975). These are persons who, for whatever reason, seem to think that their own problems, concerns, or needs are paramount. In extreme cases, the fact that a clinician is working with someone else or is in some other way busy seems incidental or even surprising to this person. These clients sometimes behave as if they expect everything else to be dropped because their matter of concern needs immediate attention.

An example of the entitled person is one who, even if the clinician is booked and has no time available, insists on being seen immediately. A patient of mine illustrated this type of behavior when he telephoned my office. My secretary, through no fault of her own, could not discourage this insistent (and persistent) person.

SECRETARY: Mr. Smith [name changed for presentation here] has called three times and insists he must speak with you right this minute.

CLINICIAN: Tell him I will try to call him back this afternoon.

SECRETARY: He already told me "no way." He says he must talk with you right now.

CLINICIAN: Okay, tell him I'm with someone, but put him through.

CLINICIAN: Hello, Mr. Smith.

CLIENT: Hi. I need to talk with you.

CLINICIAN: Mr. Smith, I wish I could talk with you now but I have two people in my office. I'll call you between 4:00 and 5:00.

CLIENT: You sound busy. Now, here's the problem . . .

Such people are difficult to work with because their emotional and intellectual makeup is such that they tend to view the world as revolving around them and their problem. Entitled clients seem to feel as if they have certain rights, and they tend to be outraged if clinicians fail to respond immediately to their wishes and desires (Edinburg et al., 1975). However, in acquiescing to these desires one runs the risk of negatively affecting other people's care or inappropriately disrupting the clinician's schedule.

There are many possible sources for such entitlement feelings, but it is beyond the scope of this book to discuss these. However, in behavioral terms, these clients' insistent methodology is reinforced in life often enough to maintain its continuation (i.e., it works). Clinicians may need to address the problem presented by such individuals because they can affect the care provided to other clients. There is no easy remedy—"entitled" individuals differ in their persistence and sensitivity. The following suggestions can be tried:

- Explain that the person cannot be seen on a "drop-in" basis because your schedule and the schedules of your other clients will not allow it.
- Just say no, you cannot talk right now but that you can call or see the client at a specified time later.
- In a setting that charges fees, offer to reserve a specific time each day for that patient. Explain that this time will be reserved and charged for whether or not it is used.
- Convey your willingness to consider helping the patient find another professional who might be more available whenever help is needed without advance notice.
- Suggest the option of seeking counseling to help remedy the underlying difficulties (see Chapter 10 for examples of how you might refer a client for help elsewhere).

These alternatives are not possible in all settings nor are they necessarily appropriate with all clients. The examples do, however, illustrate some of the different types of methods that are sometimes needed.

Another method of altering such behavior is direct counseling by a clinician. Realizing that most speech and hearing personnel are not trained in mental health counseling, there is no attempt to focus on underlying issues or etiologies of the entitled feelings. The clinician identifies and discusses with the client the types and frequencies of the intrusive behavior. Acceptable limits and appropriate goals are then established. Subsequent behavior that is within these limits is reinforced while exceptions are punished (for example, "I will not see you now, and it disappoints me that you've violated our agreement. I'll see you on Tuesday.").

There are, fortunately, relatively few clients who feel such inappropriate or extraordinary feelings of entitlement. However, when such clients are encountered, they present some very real problems for clinicians to face and try to resolve.

Insatiability

A client who appears insatiable is never really satisfied with what is occurring or what has been done. This person often demands more time, more sessions, more homework, a better hearing aid, faster progress, longer interactions with the clinician, and so forth. There are, indeed, limits to what clinicians can do. Clients who are insatiable may also feel entitled, but the two can occur independently of each other. Consider the following advice of Edinburg et al. (1975):

> *The counselor must find a way to make explicit to the [insatiable] client that his need for immediate gratification is excessive. Because the client will require some gratification, the counselor must also find a way to preserve reasonable therapeutic boundaries without causing the client undue pain. The boundaries are necessary because the counselor also knows that these clients become more anxious and guilt-ridden if they fear that these powerful impulses are uncontrollable. The demands and fears are confirmed if the counselor does not set clear limits. The counselor's ability to maintain limits and to protect himself indicate to the client that his insatiable demands can be resisted and managed.* (p. 83)

Overly Verbal

An overtalkative patient is somewhat similar to a patient who feels entitled in that such an individual can really disrupt a clinician's work schedule and even his or her personal life. Taking a phone call from an overtalkative patient at the end of the day can result in concerned, disappointed, perhaps even angry family members or friends. As Enelow and Swisher (1986) note:

> *A most difficult problem for the beginner and experienced interviewer alike is the overtalkative patient. The patient may be seen as a barrier to getting a day's work done with reasonable efficiency. He very often frustrates the clinician's efforts to get sufficient relevant information within reasonable time limits, and he is usually a major source of irritation. . . . Such a patient, then, slows down the clinician and imposes a burden of self-restraint upon him. . . . There is usually an aggressive quality to such a patient's communication which has a controlling or dominating effect. One type of over-talkative patient is the obsessional individual who insists on giving an over-detailed account, omitting nothing, not even the most trivial detail.* (p. 92)

When working with such patients, clinicians need to be careful that they are not actually encouraging them to be overly verbal. The various verbal, vocal, and nonverbal communicative encouragers and inhibitors discussed in Chapter 4 need to be carefully used and controlled. For example, clinicians want to make sure they are not unknowingly using positive head nods, forward leans or various verbal or vocal encouragers ("I see." "Uh-huh."). It may be necessary to employ some inhibiting devices such as backward leans, guggles, or interruptions. The introduction of highly closed questions, followed by a series of follow-up closed questions, can also help keep the person "on task" and less verbal than might otherwise be the case.

If clinicians have seen the person before and are aware that the individual is overly verbal, they might start the interaction with only closed questions, and rely predominantly on closed stimuli during the entire interaction. It is also a good idea to avoid scheduling such a person first in a whole day's worth of appointments!

The patient who "rambles" is also a potential problem. This person tends to talk in circles or move from point to point without apparent transitions or logical progression. Sometimes, the topics of discussion do not appear germane to the situation at hand. With such individuals, clinicians can use the various orienting devices discussed in Chapter 4. The use of summarizing or reorienting comments ("Let's get back to our discussion of _____.") are helpful in keeping the person on task, whereas the use of reflections ("So you felt that _____.") or encouragements should be avoided.

Enelow and Swisher (1986) describe another type of overly verbal client—the individual whose ververbalizations result from excessive anxiety or stress caused by the situation at hand. They suggest that friendly, reassuring, or supportive comments about the patient's fears and anxiety are often enough to reduce these tendencies to ververbalize.

Hostility

A personal anecdote is used to introduce the area of hostility. My first professional position was in a school setting, and a child was referred to me for a speech and language screening. After I had worked with the child for a few moments, it was obvious that the child's speech and language skills were considerably behind normal expectations for her age. I called the parents to discuss what I had found. After I identified myself and described my affiliation with the school, the parent responded: "If you're working for that [expletive and setting's name deleted], then you couldn't be worth a [expletive deleted] either." The parent then hung up on one very surprised new professional.

I sat back in the chair and reflected on what had just happened. It was apparent there were some feelings about the school. But was it also me? Something I said? The way I said it? Fortunately, a kind coworker was able to assure this new, surprised clinician that the child's parents were irritated with the quality of services that the child's older brother had received previously in this setting—it really wasn't me. This anecdote illustrates that the person who is subjected to someone's anger or hostility may not be the person who engendered such dissatisfaction.

A client's hostility may be the result of something that happened previously within the setting; previous interactions with an insensitive or less than fully competent professional; frustrations with or fears about a communicative difficulty; displacement of feelings toward a previously seen professional who, for example, first identified the communicative difficulty or whose prognostic suggestions did not materialize; or any number of other, often unknown, reasons. Of course, it may be the clinician who is causing hostility. The source of irritation can be discovered by probes such as the following:

"You seem a little angry at _____ ."

"I sense that you're rather irritated about _____ ."

The blanks can be filled in with whatever is appropriate (e.g., a clinician, a physician, a setting or agency, parking, certain test results, a child, the child's progress). Such probes allow clients opportunities to ventilate and release certain emotions and feelings; providing a release is one important function of interviewing and counseling.

One thing clinicians need to watch when working with hostile patients is the timing of anything they say to them. Clinicians should try to get patients to express what is on their minds and give them a full hearing before responding in any way. If clinicians respond too early or with a ready-made explanation, the full range of a patient's feelings may go unexpressed. Responding too early also appears defensive and may further fuel feelings of hostility.

Rather than deal with hostile feelings, some less-effective clinicians just ignore the situation and seem to pretend nothing is wrong. This is inappropriate because it solves nothing and can, in many cases, make matters worse. Both parties may become more angry or hostile.

Intellectualization

The term *intellectual* means using one's intelligence and reasoning abilities in a thoughtful and disciplined manner. *Intellectualization*, on the other hand, is an ego-covering defense mechanism. The person who intellectualizes is essentially talking from the head rather than from the heart. Intellectualization often conceals unresolved feelings and anguish. Consider Edinburg and associates' (1975) descriptions of an intellectualizing counseling patient:

> *The intellectualizing client has generally read several books on counseling or has avidly gleaned some knowledge of counseling from movies, friends in counseling, or other sources. This client, in telling the counselor about the problem, uses language and tone that resemble formulations being presented in a formal seminar. These presentations are without any affect and seem as though they might be about someone else. (p. 73)*

Kennedy and Charles (1990) provide another description:

> *Intellectualization refers to the manner in which some persons talk about their problems with apparent clarity and in great detail but without much emotion. They drain away their emotions by abstract-*

> *ing their problems. They do not sound [like they are resisting]*
> *because they are speaking about serious personal subjects. They are*
> *doing it at a distance, however, and the most important clue is the*
> *fact that their feelings do not seem to be present.* (p. 108)

These descriptions present a good picture of someone who is intellectualizing. There is often very little apparent emotion or feeling; there seem to be discrepancies between what these persons say and how clinicians might expect them to feel, and they often appear learned and knowledgeable.

Persons using intellectualization may expound on certain theories or beliefs (e.g., the cause of stuttering or a specific genetic syndrome), cite and describe the works of certain practitioners or researchers, or even exhibit an inordinate interest in why a disorder exists rather than what needs to be done from a remediative standpoint. Such behavior should immediately send up a flag signaling clinicians to investigate further just what the individual really knows and believes. In many cases, the person's knowledge is confined to the specific works identified. Some caution is needed with this last comment, however, because there are patients and caregivers who have appropriately read a number of sources. These persons may even be familiar with some of the more current research in the disorder area. While certainly not the major reason, this is one good reason for clinicians to keep up with a variety of literature.

Some clients who intellectualize can be difficult to deal with because they have "covered" their real feelings through the defense mechanism, and they also know just enough to be biased but not fully informed. Clinicians can rather easily assume that intellectualizing clients understand more than they really do; they may be intimidated by an appearance of being so knowledgeable, and often are thrown off by a client's apparent level of objectivity. One way of finding out how much a client actually knows is by asking questions; for example:

> "Which stuttering theory is particularly interesting to you?"
>
> "Schwartz discussed a number of ideas. Which ones were of particular interest to you?"
>
> "There are a number of language arts programs. Which ones are you thinking about?"

With both clients who are intellectualizing and those who are just well-read or intellectual, clinicians may be asked if they have read a particular book or article. The client may refer to a wide range of sources: *Reader's Digest, Psychology Today, Modern Maturity, The New England Journal of Medicine,* or even highly specialized journals in speech and hearing and related fields. It is virtually impossible to keep up with all the literature published. If you have not seen a particular item, say so. Sometimes it is useful to ask patients if they would care to share an article. When both clinician and client have read the same information, they have a common basis for discussion.

It is important to consider the potential true feelings of persons who may be intellectualizing. Intellectualization is an ego-saving reaction that helps individuals remain distant from really facing and dealing with true feelings, or the realities of some circumstances. This often occurs at subconscious levels; these individuals may be unaware that this is occurring.

Paranoia

Everyone has certain fears and concerns, and many of these are normal. Occasionally, however, clinicians encounter a patient who is exhibiting *paranoia*—the characteristics include unhealthy fears, suspicions, and feelings of persecution. Individuals exhibiting paranoia may be chronically angry, suspicious, and distrustful. They become easily convinced that other people, agencies, or institutions are against them or are out to get them. Some paranoid individuals brood, are moody, carry grudges, and are overconcerned about comments and circumstances made recently or in the past. It is common for paranoid patients to distrust the motives and intentions of clinicians and others who work with them (Enelow & Swisher, 1986).

The truly paranoid patient is rather easy to identify; such a person appears defensive when asked certain questions. Responses like "Why do you need that?" or "I don't see why that's important" are rather common. These patients may make negative comments about others in the family, other agencies, or other professionals. With a patient exhibiting paranoia, a good approach is to be consistent, low key, tactfully firm, and sensitive to topics that arouse the patient's suspicions and anger. This allows time for some trust to be built.

The clinician will also want to limit, or at least carefully use, warm and reassuring verbalizations and nonverbal behaviors because these reassurances tend to threaten some paranoid patients (Enelow & Swisher, 1986). There is a temptation to provide calm, rational explanations of the reality that contradict the paranoid feelings. However, this often can be counterproductive, at least initially, because of the strength of the ego defense that is operating. The patient's paranoia is not rationally based in the first place, so using rational arguments is essentially dealing on a different "wavelength."

Other Factors, Conditions, or Situations

Chemical Dependence

Chemical dependence, alcohol and drug abuse, are very real and pervasive problems in society. In 1991, it was estimated that 20.4 million people in the United States had a drinking problem. It was further estimated that 81.6 million family members were touched by alcohol problems (Kinney & Leaton, 1991). These figures do not include the area of illegal or prescription drug abuse. Substance use is associated with a number of communicative disorders, most commonly the effects of fetal alcohol syndrome (FAS), laryngectomy, and certain neurologic disorders.

Because of greater public awareness of the problems associated with chemical use (e.g., more stringent legal definitions of sobriety, greater penalties for substance use when driving, and various "don't drink and drive" and "sober graduation" campaigns), the percentage of motor vehicle deaths resulting from alcohol dropped from 50% in 1980 to 38% in 1989. However, alcohol continues to be a major contributor to automobile accidents, falls, drowning, burns, suicide, domestic violence, and crime in general (Kinney & Leaton, 1991).

Clinicians in many settings work with patients whose communicative disorders are related, in some way, to chemical abuse. Mills (as cited in Trace, 1995) cites several examples of ways that substance abuse affects patients:

- Some clients are subject to mood swings, disorientation, depression, erratic behavior, or violence
- People with fluency problems can experience periods of aggravated dysfluency, although some drink to calm nerves before speaking to groups
- Some depressants slow cognitive processes and cause disorientation
- Some depressants slow or alter the abilities to articulate or retrieve words efficiently

There are, as Mills points out, many other ways that speech and language skills can be affected.

Families of clients with substance abuse problems are also affected. The abuse influences how family members view each other and may be seen in reluctance to support the person who is getting speech and language assistance. Or, they may attribute everything that has happened to substance abuse. Many emotions are present in families when abuse is occurring. Mills comments that "they may feel hostility, anger, disappointment, frustration, or other emotions in response to the addiction. These emotions need to be vented and controlled before family members can be truly supportive of the patient" (as cited in Trace, 1995, p. 9). It is also possible that the effects of the abuse have numbed family members. The "family secret" is kept hidden from those outside the family and feelings are "stuffed inside." This is common among families where chemical use is occurring. Denial and minimization are also very common.

The old myth of drunks and addicts being primarily on skid row is incorrect. Only about 5% of active chemical abusers are "on the streets" (Kinney & Leaton, 1991). The large majority of individuals still function in society—going to school, holding jobs (or sometimes not holding them), paying mortgages, going to speech and hearing clinics, and so forth. A larger percentage of individuals on clinicians' caseloads is affected by chemical dependence than most professionals suspect. Clinicians should be aware of this, learn more about addiction and addictive behavior, and learn about resources to help clients (e.g., employee assistance programs, local treatment centers, Alcoholics Anonymous, Narcotics Anonymous, Cocaine Anonymous, etc.).

Grief

Individuals who are grieving generally have suffered a significant loss. They are in the process of trying to understand and adjust to a loss, and are dealing with how the loss will alter their life. Grief can be associated with death, divorce, or some other physical or emotional separation. It can also occur with the loss of communication skills that result from laryngectomy, a stroke, the onset of a hearing impairment, or some other disorder. Grief also can occur when certain diagnoses (for example, mental impairment, dysarthria, aphasia) are made or when hoped-for full recovery is not possible.

The works of Kübler-Ross (1969, 1986) dealing with grief and death, while sometimes controversial, have contributed considerably to our understanding of the grief process. She feels that *grief* is a natural, understandable process that consists of five basic stages: denial, anger, bargaining, depression, and then acceptance. Tanner's (1980) article, "Loss and Grief: Implications for the Speech-Language Pathologist and Audiologist," is a good resource on the grieving process and communicative disorders. His article is based in part on Kübler-Ross's work, and is a relatively comprehensive look at loss, the grieving process, and various implications facing speech and hearing clinicians working with those who are experiencing grief. As he notes:

• Some loss is a fundamental aspect of having or living around a disability. Patients and families can lose function (their communicative abilities) or hoped for function (the loss of hope for normal speech and language development).
• Grief is a natural and predictable reaction to loss.
• How clinicians handle patients' grief influences these persons' feelings about their disability, acceptance of the condition, motivation to get help, and desire to improve.
• Uninformed clinicians who ignore or disrupt the grief process can interfere with optimal chances for desired change. (Adapted from Tanner, 1980, p. 916.)

There are different types of loss, including real loss and symbolic loss (Tanner, 1980). Real losses include a death or separation. Symbolic losses include loss of self-esteem, stature, or some established role within a family. For example, a stroke victim may lose the position as head of the household, or a parent may lose the hope for having a college-educated child. Both types of loss—real and symbolic—are important to consider. Real or symbolic losses, or combinations of both, include the following:

• Loss of significant persons through death, divorce, or other separation (e.g., going away to college or a child of divorce moving to the other parent's home).

• Loss of external objects through some event or disaster (theft, flood, fire, bankruptcy, divorce, etc.). Intangibles such as the loss of culture, religious beliefs, or attitudes also can occur.

• Individuals moved into a nursing home may grieve over the loss of seeing and being with treasured possessions or everyday items. Tanner (1980) suggests that a mentally impaired child who is institutionalized may grieve over not having familiar toys and possessions.

• Someone with a laryngectomy may grieve over the loss of being able to swim; or an adolescent with acquired deafness may grieve over the loss of listening to a radio.

• A developmental loss, which is usually gradual and typically related to different stages in life. Examples of such losses include a child's loss of parental presence when entering kindergarten, a parent's loss as the child enters school, "losing" a child to adulthood (going away to college or into the military, or because of matrimony), losing hearing or visual acuity with age, gradual loss of memory or certain physical skills, and so forth.

• Loss of security or usual reinforcements—leaving high school or college, insecurity following a heart attack, leaving a job and beginning a new one, relocating to a far-away city, being taken out of class for speech therapy, and so forth.

• Loss of aspects of self. For example, changes in appearance following an accident or injury, or the effects of impaired memory following trauma to the brain. (Adapted from Tanner, 1980, pp. 917-920.)

The extent or severity of grief varies from that which is almost completely incapacitating to that which results in milder forms of short-term bewilderment, confusion, or depression.

Different authorities have outlined varying stages or components in the grief process. As noted earlier, Kübler-Ross (1969, 1986) talks about five stages of the grief process: (1) *denial* ("I don't believe it." "This cannot be happening." "That's not true."); (2) *anger* ("Why me?" "It isn't fair!"); (3) *bargaining* ("If I work real hard, you'll help me overcome this." "God, if you will just _____ , then I'll _____ ."); (4) *depression;* and (5) *acceptance.* Other models have also been presented. For example, Matz (1991) talks about four phases:

• *"If I deny it, it can't be true."*
• *"I have the power to undo it."* There is a feeling of power or the ability to overcome the source of grief in this phase, but it is often unrealistic. There may be hallucinations, delusions, or feelings like "If I can just see him, he would be OK" or "If he works real hard, he'll get his speech and language skills back."
• *"I can't do anything about it."* This is the point where an individual "hits bottom." Matz suggests that the patient hits bottom and, in the latter part of

the phase, begins to rebound. Realism and tentative feelings of strength or potency begin to return.

- *"I am rebuilding now and every now and then I remember."* This individual has now moved into acceptance. (Adapted from pp. 200–220.)

It is important to remember that, irrespective of which model is used (there are others not addressed here), the stages or phases of grief are not clear-cut, distinct categories. Patients do not necessarily move from one stage to another in discrete increments. Rather, it is common for clients to be working at more than one phase simultaneously, or return periodically to elements of a previous stage. In this way, the grief process can be cyclical—individuals do not necessarily move out of one phase into another and never return to a previous phase.

The amount of time it takes to move from denial to acceptance stages varies across individuals, varies in relation to the source of grief (e.g., death of a spouse or child, versus loss from theft), and differs in accordance to the closeness or importance of the loss to the individual. Tanner (1980) suggests that there are several factors that may interrupt the grieving process, including the following:

- Positively reinforcing denial
- Punishing anger that is expressed
- Bargaining with a patient
- Providing secondary gains (e.g., the individual gains special attention through grieving, which subsequently acts to perpetuate the utility of grief)
- Mood-altering drugs, such as alcohol or drugs, which act to "postpone the pain"
- Excessive distractions (e.g., immersing a patient in new activities). Patients need diversions and new activities, but not to the point that working through their feelings is ignored or postponed.
- Exhibiting anxiety about a griever's depression. Some depression is normal; excessive or extremely intense depression, however, does merit careful consideration.

Tanner also outlines the following factors that help facilitate normal grieving:

- Permit the patient to have some control (e.g., which rooms to use, time of therapy, activities used in therapy)
- Provide perspective (e.g., conveying that the pain will end and healing will occur)
- Acknowledge the reality of a loss. One clinician told a patient that the deceased pet was "only a dog and there are plenty more." Clearly, this is inappropriate and fails to acknowledge the reality of that person's loss.
- Listen to the patient. And, do not feel that certain feelings have to be explained, defended, or even condoned.

It is important to listen to patients, understand that they are hurting, acknowledge what they are saying, be supportive, and convey that the hurt will diminish and there will be better days. Clinicians frequently spend a lot of time with patients so that they can understand their clients' communicative abilities and needs. Speech-language pathologists and audiologists are not grief counselors, but they can facilitate (or impede) patients' grief processes.

Intense grief. Normal grief, particularly with the death of a loved one, can include any number of reactions such as the following:

- Physical reactions—sleeplessness, sighing and shortness of breath, digestive problems, loss of appetite, and so forth.
- Feelings of emptiness, tension, exhaustion, feeling cold, awareness of distance from others.
- Occasional preoccupation with the subject of a loss, for example, a deceased loved one.
- Occasional feelings of guilt over failing to do something, an unkind comment made, failing to say good-bye, and so forth.
- Changes in activities—restlessness, aimlessness, going somewhere and forgetting why they are there, searching for something to do, going from one thing to another without any reason, and so forth. (Adapted from Brommer, 1993, p. 108.)

Clients exhibiting excessively intense grief reactions within any of these areas, or profound personality changes (unusual euphoria, strong hostility or irritability, or severe depression), should be seen by a mental health professional with expertise in grief work. Of note, some of these reactions may occur months or even years after the actual loss occurred. Do not be fooled into thinking that something in the past is necessarily unrelated to the types of presenting symptoms seen.

Brief grief help. Many of the disorders clinicians work with involve some form of loss; helping facilitate the grief process is important. Acceptance allows patients to come to terms with certain realities and move constructively toward appropriate progress. This is not possible when someone is still denying a problem or is filled with anger. Some of the discussion in this section focuses on more intense and longer lasting grieving. However, many patients clinicians see move through the grief process quickly—sometimes in hours, days, or a week or two—particularly when clinicians are aware of what is happening and assist in expediting the process.

Crises

The term crisis is overused in everyday life—many people use it when they are busy or there are lots of things going on. However, real crises do exist for many people, and may be seen (or experienced) by audiologists and speech-language pathologists. A *crisis* is some state that exists when someone is thrown off balance emotionally by some unexpected and potentially harmful event, situation, or transition in life (Okun, 1992). The term usually refers to someone's reaction to a situation—not the situation itself (Brammer, 1993).

Okun (1992) outlines several basic types of crises that can occur:

• *Dispositional crisis*, which occurs when there is insufficient information to decide a proper course of action (e.g., which job to accept, what type of a physician to see for a particular problem, what living arrangements to choose, whether to enroll for therapy or not).

• *Anticipated life transitions*, which involve certain events or stages that occur at different age levels (e.g., changing schools, divorce, onset of a chronic or terminal illness, and so forth).

• *Traumatic stress* (e.g., rape, assault, sudden death of a loved one, sudden loss of job, accident, war, and so on).

• *Maturational or developmental crisis*, which typically relates to such issues as emotional dependence, conflicts in values, sexual identity, responses to authority, capacity for emotional intimacy, as well as problems involving self-discipline (e.g., repeatedly losing jobs because of conflicts with authority, a mid-life crisis, not being married or not having children by a certain age, intense homesickness or depression when away from home the first time, and so on).

• *Psychopathological crisis*, in which some emotional disturbance precedes and complicates a situation and, thereby, escalates it into a crisis.

• *Psychiatric emergency*, wherein the patient's overall abilities are so affected that the individual is unable to function in society without potential harm to self or others. This may be seen as a mental breakdown requiring hospitalization, or when someone is so violent that it is unsafe for that person to be in society. (Adapted from Okun, 1992, p. 214.)

A crisis is very real and, when encountered, requires help and support.

Several fundamental properties of crises are that they are typically temporary, result in considerable distress and dysfunction to the individual, involve the loss of abilities to cope well, and can have long-lasting consequences—depending on what is done and the extent to which individuals and those who are around them react (or do not react) to a crisis (Brammer, 1993). Speech and hearing clinicians typically encounter certain types of crises more than others; for example, dispositional crises are seen more than psychiatric emergencies.

The major components of working with a crisis situation include: (1) trying to help reduce tension in the other person; (2) accurately assessing the source and meaning of the stress that is occurring; (3) helping a client develop appropriate ways to respond to the situation; (4) providing emotional support, confronting denial or distorted perceptions, and helping develop appropriate cognitive perceptions (mindsets); (5) helping develop appropriate coping mechanisms, including helping facilitate the use of other resources or support networks; (6) assisting by getting the person appropriate help, if needed (e.g., family or crisis intervention specialist) (adapted from Okun, 1992, p. 218).

Threat of Suicide

A threat of suicide may occur in some settings (e.g., rehabilitations centers or extended-care facilities) more than in other settings (e.g., elementary schools). However, the threat of suicide can occur in any setting where clinicians work; and it may be something clinicians see, particularly because they are individuals with whom clients work closely and have established relationships. All threats of suicide—no matter how specifically detailed or generally referred to--are to be taken seriously. When suicide is mentioned, it can be quite disconcerting for clinicians, particularly the first time or two. The suggestions in the following paragraphs are based in large part on Meier and Davis (1993).

Any mention of suicide or self-harm should be followed up on immediately. Do not be afraid to use the word *suicide*, thinking that you are giving the other person an idea by inquiring about something that was said. If the idea has occurred to the individual, the clinician should find out whether the person has a method in mind. Meier and Davis suggest that "the more specific and concrete the method, the greater the likelihood the client will attempt suicide" (p. 43). For example, it is different if someone says, "I have a loaded gun in the car," compared to, "I'm thinking about going out and buying a gun." Another question is whether the person has attempted suicide before. This may or may not help indicate the likelihood of the person following through, but it does add potentially important insight into the possibility of committing suicide.

Take control of the situation. Someone in firm control can help to restore some order and predictability. This is not the time for indirect counseling approaches! Emphasize the positive. Sometimes expressing a positive comment becomes the "branch" that the person grabs for in deciding that suicide is not the best option. Mobilize friends, family, and caring others who can influence and stabilize the individual. Arrange, for example, for a family member to take the person home; and contact other appropriate professionals for assistance, if needed. Other resources may include a help line or a mental health professional who works within the setting. Above all, do not be afraid to act quickly and decisively. Take control rather than ignoring the warning signs of a potential suicide. Appear firm, in control, caring, supportive, and take the time necessary to handle the situation.

Concluding Comments

A number of difficult-to-deal-with client and behavior types have been described in this chapter. Because some of these have been dealt with superficially, the reader is referred to several more detailed sources; Bramson (1988), for example, has written an excellent book that focuses solely on coping with difficult people in everyday life. In the fields of medicine, psychology, counseling, and communicative disorders, there are a number of resources that contain information about dealing with difficult situations. Some examples are: Cormier and Hackney (1987), Edinburg et al. (1975), Eisenberg and Patterson (1991), Enelow and Swisher (1986), Kennedy and Charles (1990), Lavorato and McFarlane (1988), McFarlane et al. (1984), Moursund (1993), Orr and Adams (1987), and Shertzer and Stone (1980).

This chapter summarizes some of the difficult situations that professionals treating communicative disorders may encounter across their careers and offers a number of suggestions for working with such situations. There is no one perfect way of working with all of these circumstances; but using the guidelines and suggestions outlined here, the student and the professional should have a good starting point.

Chapter *10*

Ethical and Professional Matters

The work of speech-language pathologists and audiologists is important, challenging, and fulfilling. These professionals are in the unique position of being able to help provide people with the gifts of improved communicative abilities and, therefore, an improved quality of life. For this very reason, there are important responsibilities that are an integral part of clinical practice. Throughout their careers, clinicians encounter a number of different patients, patients' families and other caregivers, and disorders. They also face a number of different ethical, professional, and procedural matters that affect the delivery of clinical services. Some of these matters have been addressed throughout this book. Several other items, particularly as they relate to interviewing and counseling activities, are discussed in the sections that follow.

Extensive reference is made to the American Speech-Language-Hearing Association's (ASHA) Code of Ethics (1995b) in this chapter. However, the reader is encouraged to independently review the Code of Ethics for the matters discussed here, as well as other ethical considerations and principles. Also, sources, such as Resnick's (1993) *Professional Ethics for Audiologists and Speech-Language Pathologists* and Pannbacker, Middleton, and Vekovius' (1996) *Ethical Practices in Speech-Language Pathology and Audiology: Case Studies,* contain more extensive discussions about a number of ethical matters related to clinical practice.

Elements of Professional Practice

Key aspects of professionalism among helping professionals include having adequate knowledge of the academic discipline, developing the abilities to translate this professional knowledge into effective helping processes, being dedicated, putting the interests of the consumer ahead of personal interests, insisting on high standards of professional service to clients, and maintaining appropriate and consistent professional behavior. Professionalism involves having full qualification (i.e., knowledge and competence) and ethical integrity (Drapela, 1983; Orr & Adams, 1987).

Continuing Study

Knowledge and technology are changing constantly, and these are important factors in professional practice. The clinical worker will continue to be challenged by the need to gain and incorporate new knowledge. No matter how much we know, it is only a basis for what we will or should learn.

ASHA's Code of Ethics (Principle II-C) requires clinicians to "...continue their professional development throughout their careers" (ASHA, 1995b). Ongoing education is necessary for all clinicians in today's world, and at its heart is the desire to continue educating ourselves about the subject matter of our work. It also is vitally important as services are provided to an increasingly diverse society. To paraphrase Moursund (1993), clinicians who interview or counsel have clear choices—either continue to learn or decay; either expand knowledge or stagnate and regress.

Evaluation

Students and professionals are involved in demonstrating effectiveness of services delivered as part of service delivery accountability (Hegde & Davis, 1995; Leith, 1993). In the field of communicative disorders, there is a need to evaluate diagnostic and clinical treatment activities. There is also a need to review interviewing and counseling efforts because these are part of assessment and treatment activities. ASHA's (1995b) Code of Ethics (Principle I-G) addresses the area of evaluation in stating: "Individuals shall evaluate the effectiveness of services rendered and of products dispensed and shall only provide services or dispense products when benefit can reasonably be expected." Several other provisions of the Code of Ethics also apply to many interviewing and counseling activities:

> *Individuals shall provide all services competently.* (Principle I-A)
>
> *Individuals shall fully inform the persons they serve of the nature and possible effects of services rendered and products dispensed.* (Principle I-D)

Individuals shall not guarantee the results of any treatment or procedure, directly or by implication; however, they may make a reasonable statement of prognosis. (Principle I-F)

Individuals shall not misrepresent diagnostic information, service rendered, or products dispensed or engage in any scheme or artifice to defraud in connection with obtaining payment or reimbursement for such services or products. (Principle II-C)

Individuals' statements to the public shall provide accurate information about the nature and management of communication disorders, about the professions, and about professional services. (Principle III-D)

At a minimum, the need to provide services competently will apply to all sessions. Any or all of the preceding other provisions can apply to a given session, depending on the topics addressed.

Clinicians need to be specific and objective in their self-evaluations. This can be accomplished by thinking critically, reviewing audiotapes or videotapes of sessions, and/or using specific observational checklists or systems. The checklists in Appendices 7-A and 7-B are useful for this purpose. Other systems have been reported by Amidon (1965), Ivey (1994), McDonald and Haney (1988), Molyneaux and Lane (1982), and others. In the field of counseling, it has repeatedly been found that counselors who review videotapes of their counseling interactions gain increased confidence in their abilities and a greater awareness of the personal qualities they project during sessions. The same is true for clinicians in the fields of speech-language pathology and audiology.

Self-Representation

The ASHA Code of Ethics (Principle III-A) states: "Individuals shall not misrepresent their credentials, competence, education, training, or experience." Another provision (Principle II-B) states: "Individuals shall engage in only those aspects of the professions that are within the scope of their competence, considering their level of education, training, and experience" (ASHA, 1995b). There are several implications within these provisions.

One concern here is the possibility of patients' misconceptions about a clinician's academic degrees and areas of specialization. Writing about the practice of counseling, Edinburg, Zinberg, and Kelman (1975) note:

The counselor should not overlook misconceptions on the part of the client that have to do with his [or her] view of the counselor. If overlooked, these misconceptions, when discovered, give rise to a lack of trust in the counselor. For example, a client may address a single, female counselor with neither an M.D. nor a Ph.D. degree as "Mrs. Jones" or "Dr. Smith." It would be a mistake for the counselor to let the matter go on the assumption that the client might feel

*better being in treatment with someone who is married or who has
a more professional status. Later, when the client learned the truth,
he [or she] would be justified in feeling deceived by the counselor. A
"slip" due to misinformation on the part of the client is easily
corrected by the counselor simply stating the truth.* (p. 55)

In an unobtrusive but direct way, clinicians in such situations need to
let patients know what their correct status and salutation is.

Infrequently, the principle of misrepresentation also applies to phony
or so-called mail order degrees. For example, over the years, there have
been outfits that will supply a medical degree (M.D.) diploma for the
right price and "evidence of work or life experience." There are also
some so-called universities that will assist aspirants in gaining a Doctor
of Philosophy (Ph.D.) or Doctor of Education (Ed.D.) degree for the
right price and minimal effort. Persons with such degrees, who hold
themselves out to the public as truly being "doctors," are guilty of misrepresentation and are engaging in misleading, self-serving behavior.

Confidentiality and Patient Records

At least two provisions of the Code of Ethics apply to patient records,
appropriate access to such records, and confidentiality of these records.
These provisions are:

*Individuals shall maintain adequate records of professional ser-
vices rendered and products dispensed and shall allow access to
these records when appropriately authorized.* (Principle I-H)

*Individuals shall not reveal, without authorization, any profes-
sional or personal information about the person served professionally, unless required by law to do so, or unless doing so is necessary
to protect the welfare of the person or the community.* (Principle I-I)

Clinicians frequently interact with physicians, teachers, family members, and other speech-language pathologists or audiologists involved
with a client. Professionals may seek information from others, or information may be requested from them. The sharing of information is
appropriate and necessary, but only with the patient's knowledge and
written permission. Virtually all settings have release of information
forms to use for such permissions. The preservation of confidentiality
is an important ethical matter. The maintenance of a patient's confidentiality involves protecting all written records or tape recordings and
making sure that verbal discussions with or about clients are private
and confidential. Talking about a client in any public place has the
potential to cause big trouble.

Typically, it is useful to state the terms of confidentiality within the
setting, including who will see any information and why. It is also helpful to discuss any forms patients are asked to sign. When asking some-

one to sign an exchange of information form, be aware that individuals from a linguistically or culturally diverse background with an oral tradition can be very intimidated by such a request. Their experience in signing documents may have occurred primarily for "major life events"— weddings, death certificates, immigration, loans, and so forth. Audio- or videotape recordings also should be collected or shared only with the written permission of clients. All written or recorded materials should be protected by the rules of patient confidentiality—except in certain instances of neglect, abuse, or potential danger to the individual or others in the community that, by law, must be reported to appropriate authorities.

Human Subjects Involved in Research

Research is conducted in many settings, including university clinics, hospitals, school districts, and public and private clinics. The growth of research during the twentieth century has resulted in a dramatic increase in the number of studies involving people. Years ago, some subjects were exposed to various excessive and inappropriate risks, particularly in certain medical and psychological studies. Subjects were exposed, for example, to cancer, hepatitis, or syphilis; some were given untested drug treatments or placebo contraceptives; others were subjected to threats of electrical shock. In a number of these studies, the subjects were unaware that the research was being conducted, and they had no idea of the risks to which they were being subjected.

Today, federal and state regulations dictate a much closer review of research in most settings, particularly if patients are to be subjected to any form of physical, psychological, sociological, educational, or other risk. Common to research in all fields is a careful deliberation and approval process concerning possible risks to human subjects. Depending on the type of study and the setting, a formal approval by a responsible institution, agency, committee, or individual may be needed before any research data are collected. In the formal approval process, potential risks to subjects are carefully weighed against potential benefits to them or society. It is of particular concern that potential subjects (or their parents or caregivers) be honestly informed about the risks and benefits of their participation; that it be made clear to them that they are free to choose whether they want to participate in the study; and that they are free to withdraw from the study at any time. The anonymity of subjects also is commonly protected in all reports that result from a study.

When interviews or counseling sessions are part of either teaching efforts or research, subjects in many studies need to agree to such participation. A signed informed consent to participate is necessary for most research projects. Sources, such as Hegde (1994) and Silverman (1993), are good starting points for more information on procedures.

Key administrators in various settings (hospitals, universities, school districts, and so forth) can also help identify specific human subject policies and procedures applicable to those settings.

Note Taking and Tape Recording

Adequate records of any assessment and treatment activities are necessary in clinical practice (see ASHA, 1994; Paul-Brown, 1994), including interviewing and counseling activities. At a minimum, notes should reflect who was in attendance, primary points discussed or information shared by either party, areas of agreement or disagreement, and future activities or courses of action. Such notes should be sufficiently readable and detailed to adequately depict the session, even if needed years later. There are several potential problems with taking notes during sessions—it can create tension, be distracting, break the flow of conversation, and even lead to biased responses as interviewees take cues and adjust responses from what is being recorded (Donaghy, 1990). Thus, although necessary in many situations, the main focus during interviews and counseling sessions should not be on recordkeeping (Garrett, 1982). Rather, the emphasis should be on putting clients at ease, encouraging them to talk freely, guiding the conversation into areas and directions deemed appropriate, and interpreting the clues given by clients' words and behavior.

Taking notes should not distract from or interfere with the flow of an interview (Benjamin, 1981; Okun, 1992). Notes should be taken openly, not in hidden or secretive manners. In some cases, taking notes can convey to clients that the clinician is concerned about what is being said and is genuinely interested in the topics discussed. However, note taking should not be—and should not appear to be—used as a crutch or as an escape from interacting with interviewees.

Some form of note taking is probably beneficial for most interviewers. It is also a good idea to write more detailed case notes immediately following an interview or counseling session. Recalling the facts immediately after is a constructive alternative to disrupting a session by writing extensive notes while an interview is occurring. Laptop computers can be used to record some notes in certain settings; however, prior approval for use of one is a good idea. It is important to make sure clients are comfortable with the use of this technology. The clinician who uses a laptop computer also needs to take special care to prevent the appearance of "taking a deposition" rather than conducting an interactive interview.

With the availability of audio- and videotaping equipment, a detailed and accurate record of an interview is also possible in most clinical and educational settings. Both ways of recording client sessions are permissible, but only with prior approval. Taping another individual without his or her knowledge and consent, for whatever reason, is inappropriate.

Discussing Fees

The need to discuss fees and payments for services does not occur within some settings—Head Start programs, schools, and other publicly or privately supported settings that do not charge fees. The subject of fees does come up within most other settings such as hospitals, private and community-based clinics, and most university speech and hearing clinics.

Some clinicians feel uncomfortable discussing fees with clients, so these types of discussions are often relegated to a clinic secretary, the business office, or a university supervisor. Discussing fees with clients is important, whether they are paying the entire fee for the services themselves or they are being partially or fully reimbursed by a third party (e.g., private or public insurance, a relative, or an employer).

Clinicians should provide clients with complete price and fee information prior to rendering actual services. People need to know what they will be charged for the services to be provided. When appropriate, it is the professional's responsibility to discuss fees in an honest, forthright, and knowledgeable manner. For students, discussing fees may or may not be appropriate, depending on the policies of the university clinic or the site of an internship. A supervisor, clinic secretary, or clinic director should be consulted before a student discusses fees with clients.

Making Referrals

A clinician making a referral transfers the client to another professional who is more able, through specialization or experience, to provide the specific service needed by the client (Shertzer & Stone, 1980). By referring a client elsewhere, the clinician is attempting to serve the client's best interests. Examples of a referral might be for a medical consultation, special education evaluation, psychological or psychiatric evaluation, or it might even be for services from another communicative disorders professional who has greater expertise or resources for assisting with the problem at hand. The Code of Ethics (ASHA, 1995b) states: "Individuals shall use every resource available, including referral when appropriate, to ensure that high quality service is provided" (Principle I-B).

The sincere, secure professional is aware of the need for, and is comfortable making, appropriate referrals to other specialists. Such an individual is not afraid to make a recommendation when it is in the best interests of a client. Clients are more likely to accept and act on referrals when clinicians give clear and straightforward, but tactful, reasons for their recommendation. The following are several useful guidelines for referrals that have been adapted from MacLean and Gould (1988) and Sweeney (1971):

1. If possible, be personally acquainted and familiar with the professionals or agencies you are suggesting. Become familiar with services within your community.

2. Discuss the reasons for suggesting the referral with clients.

3. Describe for clients the types of information and areas of concern that they should share with the professional or agency to whom individuals are being referred.

4. Everyone involved should have a clear understanding about any information that will be shared between clinicians and other professionals or agencies, and how this sharing will be accomplished (e.g., by mailed report or by telephone call).

Referrals to other speech and hearing professionals who are out of the area or out of state can be made through the use of the American Speech-Language-Hearing Association's *Guide to Professional Services in Speech-Language Pathology and Audiology,* the *ASHA Directory,* or various state association directories. All of these resources are updated periodically.

Lavorato and McFarlane (1988) note that some clients balk at seeing another type of specialist, particularly a psychologist, psychiatrist, or other mental health professional. Resistance may occur because of the stigma attached; anticipated cost; or simply frustration, anger, or confusion about being referred elsewhere. They suggest four ways to make such a referral. One way is to calmly but directly recommend that the client "consult with" or "talk with" another specialist. Terms such as "consider psychotherapy" or "be evaluated by" should not be used; rather, the words "talk with" are more casual and nonthreatening. A second method is to use the terms "counseling" or "counselor" rather than "psychotherapist" or "psychologist." Lavorato and McFarlane's third suggestion is to use descriptive phrases such as "see a specialist who can help with problems like you are experiencing." Their fourth suggestion is to use the client's own statements as a springboard for the form of the recommendation. Lavorato and McFarlane (1988) provide the following examples:

> CLIENT: *Seeing you is like getting psychotherapy.*
>
> CLINICIAN: *I'm glad our sessions are helping you. Have you considered seeing a specialist in psychotherapy?*
>
> CLIENT: *I'm so upset. I don't know how I'll handle this problem.*
>
> CLINICIAN: *I'm sensing that the problem preoccupies you. That burden could be relieved by seeing a counselor. I'd like to suggest that* _____ . (pp. 252-253)

Many needs for referral are relatively obvious, particularly when they are related to medical issues. However, it is sometimes a little less clear-cut when there is a need for psychological forms of counseling. The information in Chapter 7 should be helpful in determining the need for a referral. Other sources of information include Clark (1994b), Leith (1993), Luterman (1991), Rollin (1987), and Stone and Olswang (1989).

Referrals for some individuals from linguistically or culturally different cultures may require special consideration. What, for example, a clinician interprets as interpersonal resistance may actually have its base in cultural values. Or, there may be logistic problems some clinicians fail to consider. For example, as Zuniga (1992) writes:

> *Does the family have transportation for following through with a referral you make? They may gladly agree with all your plans but be embarrassed to inform you that they have no means of transportation or they may not know how to traverse freeways that you assume everyone can negotiate.* (p. 173)

With certain patients, particularly newer immigrants, it may be necessary to accompany them to be a model on the use of elevators, to help with office protocol, to help interpret, or for comforting purposes.

Reliability and Validity

Reliability and validity are important concepts in the scientific method, and they apply to various clinical activities. In interviewing and counseling, *reliability* is the gaining of the same or consistent results at different times. *Validity* is the degree to which information appears to be true. It is important for clinicians to consider the reliability and validity of information obtained in interviews. A positive relationship between the information obtained on a written case history, behavior observed, and information collected during interviewing and counseling sessions should be apparent if clinicians are to accept the data as being reliable. Thus, a comparison of the information gathered across these three situations is a good check on the consistency and the accuracy of the information.

The deliberate distorting, withholding, or fabricating of information is not usually a concern in most settings because clients have sought help and are motivated to be honest and cooperative. The primary exceptions here are certain malingerers, certain insurance reimbursement frauds, or certain defensive reactions (including defense mechanisms). However, in the absence of these problems, remember that a clinical or educational environment may be uncomfortable or unfamiliar to some interviewees and certain areas of discussion may be very sensitive. Thus, a client's written and verbal accounts and the behavior a clinician observes may not be fully consistent.

There are a number of ways to check the validity of an oral report. Clinicians can ask themselves the following questions before accepting information at face value:

1. Can the information be verified or reproduced?
2. Is there adequate and reliable information available?
3. Does the information come from several different sources?
4. Does the information gathered from records, from testing, and from background information correspond with the results of an interview?

5. Does the information correspond with our professional judgment and with the opinions of others?
6. Does the client provide information freely, quickly, and without obvious reluctance or hesitation? Of course, such a free and speedy provision of information is based on having adequate skills in the language used during an interaction.

When clinicians rely primarily or exclusively on closed-ended questions, it is particularly difficult to determine the validity or truthfulness of the client's responses (Enelow & Swisher, 1986; Shipley & Wood, 1996). When using closed questions, clinicians should consider the level of information that is requested within each question, the social acceptability of the information asked for, and the response choices the questions allow. For example, if a clinician were to ask parents about their methods of discipline at home, some parents might be reluctant to share this information out of fear that the interviewer would find their approaches unacceptable. Such hesitation may be seen with some clients, including those from linguistically and culturally diverse backgrounds, who view a clinician as operating in a judgmental fashion.

There is another way to look at clients' responses. That is, any response a clinician receives—whether accurate or inaccurate—is valid if clinicians consider it from the viewpoint that it reveals where the client dares to be honest and trustworthy with them at that point in time. In other words, there may be an important reason why an interviewee is not completely honest. In such cases, the clinician should note the level of concern or anxiety in an interviewee and, at some point, consider exploring the subject openly.

When discrepancies occur in an interview, they should not be ignored (Darley, 1978). The information or behavior in question should be verified unobtrusively at a later point, either during the same interview or on another occasion. Except when confrontation techniques are needed for some reason, blunt challenges to the veracity of information provided by the interviewee are typically avoided whenever possible.

Finally, as noted in Chapter 4, clinicians should remember that agreement does not necessarily mean information is accurate or valid. An entire family or group may agree on something, but that does not mean their perceptions are necessarily accurate. Remember, at one time in history, almost everyone "knew" the world was flat; the sources of this information were reliable (i.e., consistent) but the information simply was not valid.

Being Culturally Aware

The United States is changing demographically at a very fast rate. It is a country whose population is growing older and living longer. It is also growing more ethnically and culturally diverse (see Chapter 8). About

50 percent of ASHA members provide services to individuals who do not speak English as their native language (ASHA, 1993). In many cities, English is not the most prevalent language and/or a large number of languages and dialects may be spoken.

The importance of culture was described in Chapter 3 and again in Chapter 8. To work effectively with a diverse population, it is critical to learn about the various cultures and their values and traditions. Clinicians have a responsibility to learn about the backgrounds of their clients so that they are more aware of and sensitive to the differences among people from different cultures. Effective cross-cultural practice is enhanced when clinicians are able to identify and accept, in a nonjudgmental way, alternative ways of viewing the world (Sue, 1988).

There are several things that culturally effective clinicians avoid doing. They avoid imposing their own values and expectations onto clients from different cultural backgrounds; they avoid stereotyping and applying overall group generalities onto specific clients; and they appropriately modify their activities with individual clients and families. For learning more about working effectively across various cultures, the following sources are highly recommended: Battle (1993a), Lee and Richardson (1991), Paniagua (1994), Pederson (1985), Pederson, Draguns, Lonner, and Trimble (1989), Pederson and Ivey (1993), Roseberry-McKibbin (1995), and Sue (1988).

Avoiding Discrimination

ASHA's Code of Ethics (Ethical Proscription I-C) states: "Individuals shall not discriminate in the delivery of professional services on the basis of race or ethnicity, gender, age, religion, national origin, sexual orientation, or disability" (ASHA, 1995b). Discrimination of any of these types is obviously unethical, inappropriate, and in many cases, illegal.

One form of discrimination that some clinicians may be unaware of relates to Section 504 of the Rehabilitation Act of 1973. This law was passed to end many types of discrimination against disabled persons. Basically, the law prohibits discrimination against individuals with disabling conditions by mandating that "any program or activity of a recipient of federal financial assistance cannot discriminate against handicapped [sic] people." Thousands of hospitals, public elementary and high schools, colleges and universities, and other facilities receive federal assistance of some form and, therefore, fall under Section 504's provisions.

Using hospitals and the hearing impaired as examples, services provided to hearing and hearing-impaired clients must be provided equally. To ensure that equal service and levels of patient knowledge are provided, the hospital may be required to provide a telecommunication device for the deaf (TDD), a qualified interpreter, or other services that will ensure that equal and appropriate services are available. Appropriate adaptations are also needed in many other educational and clinical settings to ensure equal treatment for individuals who are deaf, hard-of-hearing, or blind, or who have cerebral palsy, mental impairment, or other types of physical or mental disabilities. Further information and guidelines are available from the U.S. Department of Health and Human Services or the appropriate departments dealing with civil rights in the various states. The National Center for Law and the Deaf, a public service of Gallaudet College in Washington, DC, also prepares excellent explanations of this and other laws as they pertain to deafness and hearing impairment.

Criticism of Other Professionals

It is not unusual for the clinician to encounter clients, or the family members and caregivers of clients, who have sought the advice of several different professionals. Consequently, these clients may have, on occasion, received varied and conflicting information. When asked about the logic or accuracy of another professional's opinion, clinicians need to be very careful not to criticize or second guess others. Typically, it is best for clinicians to limit discussion to their own direct observations and the information they have collected. Some awkward situations can be handled by pointing out differences in the times or dates of previous testing (such as testing done several years ago versus today), or differences resulting from the different test environments or procedures used. Clinicians may also need to inform clients that differing opinions exist about certain disorders. Within the field, there can be several schools of thought about disorders and treatments, each of which can lead to positive clinical results.

Even when clinicians do not approve of or agree with another opinion, they should still be careful not to criticize another professional. Rather, a positive approach is typically much more effective (Hartbauer, 1978; McFarlane, Fujiki, & Brinton, 1984). Clinicians can present the rationale for their conclusions and recommendations and be willing to suggest or discuss alternative courses. If the logic of a clinician's thinking is followed by the client on a step-by-step basis, there is usually no need to defend any recommendations made or to criticize others. Although it is sometimes tempting to criticize the work of another person, particularly when inadequate services were provided, such criticisms rarely do anything positive except make the criticizer feel superior for a couple of moments. And, as the adage goes, "what goes around comes around." The wise clinician is well aware that criticism of someone else rarely accomplishes anything positive and often has long-lasting negative consequences!

Inappropriate Personal Relationships

Clinicians are warned, as are practitioners in other helping professions, against involvement in inappropriate personal relationships. It is not unusual for a clinician to be attracted to a client or to a family member or caregiver of a client. Such attraction is in human nature—it is normal and certainly nothing for a clinician to feel guilty about (Enelow & Swisher, 1986). However, for a clinician to take action on such an interest or desire is usually inappropriate and it can have very negative, long-term consequences for all parties. The incidence and problems associated with inappropriate personal relationships are discussed more frequently in fields such as medicine, psychiatry, psychology, and counseling (Biggs & Blocher, 1987; Edinburg, Zinberg, & Kelman, 1975; Enelow & Swisher, 1986; Moursund, 1993). The issue of sexual involvement emanating from the workplace has surfaced more in these other fields than in the field of communicative disorders. However, although neither well publicized nor typically mentioned in literature, these situations do occur in this field; and they are more likely to occur in long-term treatment relationships. Professionals have lost their jobs and even their careers over such indiscretions; and some have ended up in court over difficulties resulting from inappropriate personal relationships. Careers—after years of education and practice—have been totally destroyed because of inappropriate relationships with others. Of course, this does not even begin to address the effects on a client or on a client's significant other, children, other family members and friends. It is certainly wise for clinicians to consider long-range consequences and implications before engaging in such relationships. Friendships and social relationships with clients or their caregivers, no matter how platonic, are seldom wise (Orr & Adams, 1987).

Terminating Clinical Services

Providing closure means wrapping things up appropriately. More frequently, clinicians use the term terminating. As soon as the word *terminating* is used, it is likely some readers have some form of a negative reaction. Termination is a word that seems to engender the same types of negative feelings as do these terms: statistics, test, masters comps, or the Internal Revenue Service. Moursund (1993) writes eloquently about the concept of termination in our culture:

> *It is a hallmark of our culture that we are reluctant to talk openly about ending relationships or cutting off contact. We say "see you later" instead of "goodbye" and disguise the finality of long-term partings (graduations, moving away) with promises to keep in touch. Even death, that most final of endings, is referred to as passing on, and Western religion is replete with reassurances that important relationships need not end—that, in the words of the old*

hymn, "we shall meet in the sweet bye-and-bye." Ending a meaning-
ful relationship is unpleasant if not downright painful; none of us
likes to give up something we care about. It is easier to pretend that
it will not happen, that it is not happening, that it did not happen,
and then deal with the reality later, when we have found new
friends and new interests and the pain of parting has had time to
subside. It is a great temptation to clients and therapists (being,
after all, people like everyone else) to treat their endings in the same
way: to ignore the fact that termination is coming, to disguise its
reality with pseudo-plans to meet again in one way or another, or
to slide through the last sessions without knowing that they will, in
fact, be the last. (p. 91)

Termination, particularly from ongoing treatment, can be difficult
for both clinicians and clients unless clinicians have planned for it, and
prepared their clients and themselves for this ending. Remember that in
a helping profession, it is the clinician's obligation to provide the quick-
est and most efficient clinical services possible (MacLean & Gould, 1988).
The termination of an ongoing relationship should be discussed, at least
periodically, throughout the course of a therapeutic relationship (Hackney & Cormier, 1994; Moursund, 1993). With regard to counseling, it has
been said that the stage for termination begins to be set during an initial
interview as a working agreement for meeting the treatment goals is
established (Edinburg et al., 1975). Although this does not always happen, clinicians do need to prepare their clients (and themselves) throughout the course of service delivery for the day when clinical services
will no longer be needed. When the day does come, the client should
understand why—for example, because the goals have been met or because no additional progress appears possible.

When a relationship terminates, the actual parting is sometimes sad
and emotionally trying. Some clients and clinicians may even go through
a form of grieving because, in essence, a loss is occurring. The other
party will no longer be seen on an ongoing basis. It is like the sadness
many parents experience when their sons or daughters leave home. At
parting, one or both of the parties may experience a variety of emotions—anger, fear, guilt, or a sense of loss (Moursund, 1993). These are
natural reactions that need to be acknowledged. However, Moursund
(1993) also notes that clinicians can and should feel good about the
progress made and accomplishments gained. In effect, clinicians can
feel good that they "put themselves out of a job" because of a job well
done.

There are some specific considerations clinicians should keep in
mind when terminating a clinical relationship. Any loose ends should
be tied up and, in that regard, the termination timed wisely and appropriately. A clinician should also consider whether any referrals are appropriate for follow-up care or for treatment of any other problems. In
terminating a relationship, clinicians should attempt to "keep the door

open" so their client feels free to contact them with any future questions or concerns (McDonald & Haney, 1988). It is also a good idea for clinicians to follow up on their clients after termination. Most clients truly appreciate a call sometime later just to make sure they are doing well and everything is OK. Clinicians also feel good knowing that their patients have maintained any progress made, when this is the case.

Risk Management Strategies

There is a certain element of risk in all human service activities, including speech-language pathology and audiology. These fields are not considered to have "catastrophic exposure" (ASHA, 1994), but legal action is brought against practitioners from time to time. A majority of these actions involve questions about improper assessment or treatment, hearing aid dispensing, employment conflicts, physical injuries, and improper diagnosis. Less frequent legal actions have involved sexual harassment, property damage, failure to provide sufficient information to clients, and false guarantees of results (ASHA, 1994). Many areas of litigation involve discussions with others in areas of assessment and treatment, which often involve interviewing and counseling interactions.

ASHA (1994) has identified six general areas—awareness and education of the practitioner, effective communication, documentation, confidentiality, informed consent, and client safety—of exposure to risks of conduct (see Table 10.1). Problems in these areas can result in legal and ethical difficulties. In reviewing ASHA's risk areas, notice that many of these items have been addressed in the context of interviewing and counseling within this chapter or throughout the book.

Dealing with Failures

Sir James M. Barrie reportedly said, "We are all failures—at least the best of us are" (MacLean & Gould, 1988, p. 43). As hard as it may be to admit, there are some people a clinician simply cannot help. Some clients may not mesh well with a clinician's personality or may not be willing to enter into a helper-helpee relationship. Being honest about this possibility is a sign of wisdom and clinical maturity.

No one should expect to succeed all the time. As Kennedy and Charles (1990) comment, interviewers and counselors who cannot accept their own limitations and at least occasional defeats are probably in the wrong line of work. No clinician is immune to the experience of failure. In a professional field, clinicians expect to succeed and be able to help—but this is not always possible. In their book, *The Imperfect Therapist,* Kottler and Blau (1989) point out that professionals in the helping professions can be their own worst enemies if they do not acknowledge self-doubts, or if they fail to realize when they are in

TABLE 10.1 Six Areas of Exposure to Risks of Conduct and Methods of Reducing These Risks

1. Awareness and Education of Practitioner
   - Identify potential risks.
   - Eliminate or reduce risks by providing an accepted standard of care.
   - Practice within the scope of your professional competence, licensure, and certification.
   - Use only licensed or registered titles.
   - Stay current with developments in your profession.
   - Keep abreast of evolving standards of practice.
   - Maintain professional competence through continuing education.
   - Know state licensing laws.
   - Know applicable codes of ethics.
   - Know relevant scopes of practice.
   - Know and use current preferred practice patterns, guidelines, and position statements.
   - Use only equipment and test materials with which you are trained or knowledgeable.
   - Refer when you do not possess the knowledge, expertise, and credentials to provide a needed service.
   - Be certain of licensure, certification, and other qualifications of all persons to whom referrals are made, as well as those of employers or employees.
   - Know and use the policies and procedures of the hospital or organizations with which you are employed.

2. Effective Communication
   - Establish a positive relationship with clients.
   - Be a good listener.
   - Explain test results, treatment goals, treatment plans, and procedures, as well as realistic outcomes.
   - Take time to explain answers in lay terms.
   - Avoid making statements that mislead clients into unreasonable expectations.
   - Address both benefits and limitations of products or treatment.
   - Encourage observation of procedures by caregivers.
   - Make full disclosure of fees, billing schedules, and arrangements for missed sessions before treatment begins or equipment is dispensed.
   - Provide written warranties and disclaimers of guarantees.
   - Secure signature of client, caregiver, or significant other to acknowledge transfer and indicate understanding of written warnings, warranties, and disclaimer of guarantees.

3. Documentation—Record Keeping and Reporting
   - Be aware that the care with which documents are kept will reflect the quality of care clients receive, and that these documents may be subpoenaed.
   - Make all entries accurate, thorough, and legible.
   - When corrections are necessary:
     - Never "white out" or obliterate;
     - Draw a line through incorrect information;

(Continued)

TABLE 10.1 *(Continued)*

        - Initial and date the correction; and
        - Note why the correction was necessary.
- Document all personal and telephone contacts with client and family.
- Keep copies of all correspondence with or about the client.
- Document all contacts with other professionals regarding the client.
- Document failure to show, cancellation, or rescheduling of appointments.
- Document noncompliant behavior by describing behavior that leads to that opinion, rather than making judgmental or opinionated statements.
- Document limitations of treatment progress.
- Document recommendations.
- If team recommendations differ from your own, document your own recommendations and state rationale and conclusions.
- Keep records of all dispensed products.
- Keep records of equipment maintenance and calibration.
- Document warnings or dangers of products.
- Document informed consent for evaluation and treatment procedures.
- Document consent for dispensing or receiving client information.
- Document when and where all client information was sent.

4. Confidentiality
   - Release to a specific entity only information that was requested in writing.
   - Obtain a signed and witnessed release.
   - Know who is authorized to view or receive records by awareness of:
        - State regulations;
        - Policies and procedures of hospitals or organizations with which you are affiliated;
        - The client's rights of access to records;
        - Provider's right of reasonable restrictions on access.
   - Document does not have to be provided at any time or any place requested by the client, but must be provided at a mutually agreed-on time and place.
   - Provider may need information to be available to explain or interpret information.
   - Provider can charge reasonable fees for copies.
   - Use fax or other forms of electronic mail cautiously to prevent disclosure to unauthorized individuals.

5. Informed Consent
   - Obtain informed consent for evaluation and treatment procedures.
   - Inform the client of the following elements to obtain a valid informed consent:
        - Nature of ailment, proposed treatment, risk, consequences of treatment;
        - Probability of success;
        - Treatment alternatives; and
        - Prognosis.
   - Determine who has the authority to sign an informed consent by securing knowledge of:
        - State laws for determining minor status;

TABLE 10.1 *(Continued)*

- State and local laws for determining legal guardian for minors in the absence of a parent; and
- Policies and procedures of the hospital or organization with which you are affiliated.
- Treat minors only when accompanied by a parent or guardian or when written permission has been obtained to treat in their absence.

6. Client Safety
   - Make sure physical environment is free of hazards.
   - Structure activities to reduce client injury.
   - Follow universal infection control procedures.
   - Ensure the availability of emergency services based on evaluation and treatment risks.

Source: American Speech-Language-Hearing Association (1994, March). Professional liability and risk management for the audiology and speech-language pathology professions. *Asha,* 36 (Supplement 12), 31–32. Copyright 1994 by and presented here with permission of the American Speech-Language-Hearing Association, Rockville, MD.

trouble. Kottler and Blau also remind us that failures can be useful in that, if properly understood, they help clinicians improve their future performance. Van Riper (1966) conveys similar thoughts in his classic article "Success and Failure in Speech Therapy." A clinician's growth is related to finding out what works well, recognizing what does not work well, and trying to discover why.

Concluding Comments

This chapter discusses a number of topics dealing with ethical and professional matters. There are undoubtedly many additional areas that are unique to specific settings and cases. In some settings, procedure and policy manuals are available to specify how certain matters should be handled. In other cases, the reader may want to review sources such as ASHA's Code of Ethics (ASHA, 1995b), the "Scope of Practice" article (ASHA, 1990), or "Preferred Practice Patterns for the Professions..." (ASHA, 1993); consult with peers or supervisors; and use good sense. Always, though, the clinician should consider what is best for the client and what is the professional thing to do.

Chapter *11*

A Few Final Thoughts

Interviewing and counseling with individuals, families, and other caregivers is an important and rewarding aspect of practice. It provides wonderful opportunities to get to know people better, and to serve the needs of those impacted by a communicative disorder. When clinicians interview and counsel well, they provide substantial help to others and find these activities very fulfilling.

Learning to interview and counsel—or improving skills and abilities in these areas—involves acquiring basic knowledge and skills, observation, practice, and experience. Formal instruction in interviewing and counseling, such as through a class, is certainly highly advantageous. Unfortunately, as noted several times in this book, undergraduate and graduate-level coursework in interviewing and counseling with communicative disorders is often inadequate (Clark, 1994a; Colton & Casper, 1990; Johnson, 1994).

Several years ago, Culpepper, Mendel, and McCarthy (1994) surveyed all American Speech-Language-Hearing Association-accredited university programs and reported that, at a majority of universities, less than 25% of graduates had even taken a course in counseling. Only 17% of the respondants at these universities felt that graduates were adequately prepared to meet the counseling needs of communicatively disordered clients. This certainly parallels Gregory's (1995) suggestion that many students and professional clinicians comment on never having had a course in counseling, or do not recognize when counseling was covered in a course. So, students who are attending a school that offers such coursework should take advantage of it. The knowledge will be important in professional practice.

Students in programs that do not have interviewing and counseling coursework and practicum available, or professionals who have completed their preprofessional education without such exposure, should consider taking at least a foundational course in this area. Often coursework in interviewing and counseling is available in disciplines such as counseling, psychology, regular or special education, social work, or other education- or health-related disciplines.

Other helpful sources of information include attending workshops or seminars and reading various materials about interviewing and counseling, either in communicative disorders or more general works in these areas. These forms of instruction provide the basic principles of interviewing and counseling. Several readable and useful resources about interviewing and counseling in general include:

Donaghy, W. G. (1990). *The interview: Skills and applications.* Salem, WI: Sheffield.
Garrett, A. (1982). I*nterviewing: Its principles and methods* (3d ed.). New York: Family Service Association of America.
Ivey, A. E. (1994). *Intentional interviewing and counseling: Facilitating client development in a multicultural society* (3d ed.). Pacific Grove, CA: Brooks/ Cole.
Meier, S. T., & Davis, S. R. (1993). *The elements of counseling* (2d ed.). Pacific Grove, CA: Brooks/Cole.
Okun, B. F. (1992). *Effective helping: Interviewing and counseling techniques* (4th ed.). Pacific Grove, CA: Brooks/Cole.
Pederson, P. B., & Ivey, A. E. (1993). *Culture-centered counseling and interviewing skills: A practical guide.* Westport, CT: Praeger.
Shipley, K. G., & Wood, J. M. (1995). *The elements of interviewing.* San Diego: Singular Publishing Group.
Stewart, C. J., & Cash, W. B. (1994). *Interviewing principles and practices* (7th ed.). Dubuque, IA: William C. Brown.

Several useful resources for interviewing and counseling related specifically to the field of communicative disorders include:

Andrews, J. R., & Andrews, M. A. (1990). *Family based treatment in communicative disorders: A systemic approach.* Sandwich, IL: Janelle Publications.
Bloom, C. M., & Cooperman, D. K. (1992). *The clinical interview: A guide for speech-language pathologists and audiologists* (2d ed.). Rockville, MD: National Student Speech-Language-Hearing Association.
Clark, J. G., & Martin, F. N. (1994). *Effective counseling in audiology: Perspectives and practice.* Englewood Cliffs, NJ: Prentice-Hall.
Luterman, D. M. (1991). *Counseling the communicatively disordered and their families* (2d ed.). Austin, TX: Pro-Ed.
Rollin, W. J. (1987). *The psychology of communication disorders in individuals and their families.* Englewood Cliffs, NJ: Prentice-Hall.
Schum, R. L. (1986). *Counseling in speech and hearing practice.* Rockville, MD: National Student Speech-Language-Hearing Association.
Webster, E. J., & Ward, L. M. (1993). *Working with parents of young children with disabilities.* San Diego, CA: Singular Publishing Group.

Other useful works are listed in the References at the end of this book.

Observing interviewing and counseling situations bolsters an understanding of the principles described in this book, from the books listed on the previous page, from coursework, or from workshops or seminars. Observing interviewing and counseling sessions can be particularly useful when the session is being conducted by an experienced, skilled practitioner. It is less helpful to observe individuals who are just learning or are "less effective" interviewers or counselors. By observing others in clinical settings, students and professionals can improve their understanding of the various techniques available and the many situations and reactions that can occur. Clinicians in communicative disorders also can benefit by observing skilled practitioners in other disciplines.

Observation can be done in person (either in the room or through observation windows) or by videotape. Audiotapes of particular situations are beneficial in some circumstances, but many nonverbal behaviors and interchanges cannot be observed this way. Using some type of checklist or observational system when observing is recommended. This helps provide structure and purpose to what is being observed because observers focus on specific techniques or factors in the interchange. Two such methods are in Appendices 7-A and 7-B. Amidon (1965), Ivey (1994), McDonald and Haney (1988), Molyneaux and Lane (1982), Shipley (1992), and others report on other useful methods.

Academic preparation and observation provide a base of knowledge and understanding, but practice and "on-line" interviewing and counseling experience are also necessary. In the field of communicative disorders, everyone who has progressed from early academic coursework into clinical practicum is aware that taking coursework or reading about something is different from actual clinical service. Exposure to information is the basis of knowledge, but applying this information to patients and caregivers often is a different story. Clinicians learn to effectively assess and treat different communicative disorders through a combination of academic knowledge and direct experience. Similarly, effective interviewers and counselors learn by doing. Practice allows clinicians to solidify their basic knowledge and understanding, directly experience the effects of using different approaches and techniques, determine the most effective techniques for different situations, and refine the myriad of skills and abilities needed to interview and counsel competently and confidently.

As noted in Chapter 10, clinicians need to continue developing and refining abilities and skills throughout their careers. Clinicians will continue to learn more about interviewing and counseling and different communicative disorders from new experiences with clients, from the study of new research articles and books, from participation in professional conferences, and so forth.

Finally, enjoy the process of interviewing and counseling and the opportunities to interact with others during these interactions. Interviewing and counseling activities are richly rewarding, enjoyable, and highly beneficial aspects of professional service.

APPENDIX A

CHILD CASE HISTORY FORM

General Information

Child's Name: _____ Date of Birth: _____

Address: _____ Phone: _____

City: _____ Zip: _____

Does the child live with both parents? _____

Mother's Name: _____ Age: _____

Mother's Occupation: _____ Business Phone: _____

Father's Name: _____ Age: _____

Father's Occupation: _____ Business Phone: _____

Referred By: _____ Phone: _____

Address: _____

Pediatrician: _____ Phone: _____

Address: _____

Family Doctor: _____ Phone: _____

Address: _____

Brothers and Sisters (include names and ages):

_____

_____

_____

_____

What languages does the child speak? What is the child's primary language?

What languages are spoken in the home? What is the primary language spoken?

With whom does the child spend most of his or her time?

Source: From Kenneth G. Shipley and Julie G. McAfee, *Assessment in Speech-Language Pathology: A Resource Manual,* pp. 14–21. Copyright 1992 by and reprinted with permission of Singular Publishing Group, San Diego, CA.

Describe the child's speech-language problem.

How does the child usually communicate (gestures, single words, short phrases, sentences)?

When was the problem first noticed? By whom?

What do you think may have caused the problem?

Has the problem changed since it was first noticed?

Is the child aware of the problem? If yes, how does he or she feel about it?

Have any other speech-language specialists seen the child? Who and when? What were their conclusions or suggestions?

Have any other specialists (physicians, psychologists, special education teachers, etc.) seen the child? If yes, indicate the type of specialist, when the child was seen, and the specialist's conclusions or suggestions.

Are there any other speech, language, or hearing problems in your family? If yes, please describe.

Prenatal and Birth History

Mother's general health during pregnancy (illnesses, accidents, medications, etc.).

Length of pregnancy: _____   Length of labor: _____

General condition: _____   Birth weight: _____

Circle type of delivery: head first   feet first   breech   caesarian

Were there any unusual conditions that may have affected the pregnancy or birth?

Medical History

Provide the approximate ages at which the child suffered the following illness and conditions:

Allergies _____	Asthma _____	Chicken Pox _____
Colds _____	Convulsions _____	Croup _____
Dizziness _____	Draining Ear _____	Ear Infections _____
Encephalitis _____	German Measles _____	Headaches _____
High Fever _____	Influenza _____	Mastoiditis _____
Measles _____	Meningitis _____	Mumps _____
Pneumonia _____	Seizures _____	Sinusitis _____
Tinnitus _____	Tonsillitis _____	Other _____

Has the child had any surgeries? If yes, what type and when (e.g., tonsilectomy, adenoidectomy, etc.)?

Describe any major accidents or hospitalizations.

Is the child taking any medications? If yes, identify.

Have there been any negative reactions to medications? If yes, identify.

Developmental History

Provide the approximate age at which the child began to do the following activities:

Crawl _____   Sit _____   Stand _____

Walk _____   Feed self _____   Dress self _____

Use toilet _____

Use single words (e.g., *no, mom, doggie,* etc.): _____

Combine words (e.g., *me go, daddy shoe,* etc.): _____

Name simple objects (e.g., *dog, car, tree,* etc.): _____

Use simple questions (e.g., *Where's doggie?* etc.): _____

Engage in a conversation: _____

Does the child have difficulty walking, running, or participating in other activities that require small- or large-muscle coordination?

Are there or have there ever been any feeding problems (e.g., problems with sucking, swallowing, drooling, chewing, etc.)? If yes, describe.

Describe the child's response to sound (e.g., responds to all sounds, responds to loud sounds only, inconsistently responds to sounds, etc.).

Educational History

School: _____   Grade: _____

Teacher(s): _____

How is the child doing academically (or preacademically)?

Does the child receive special services? If yes, describe.

How does the child interact with others (e.g., shy, aggressive, uncooperative, etc.)?

If enrolled for special education services, has an Individualized Educational Plan (IEP) been developed? If yes, describe the most important goals.

Provide any additional information that might be helpful in the evaluation or remediation of the child's problem.

Person completing form: _____

Relationship to child: _____

Signed: _____   Date: _____

APPENDIX B

EXAMPLE OF A DISORDER-SPECIFIC CASE HISTORY FORM
[FOR ADULT VOICE CASES]

Background and Identifying Information

Name: _____ Date of Birth: _____ Age: _____ Sex: _____

Occupation: _____ Current Date: _____

Home Address: _____

Home Telephone: _____ Work Telephone: _____

Referred by: _____ Phone: _____

Primary Physician: _____ Phone: _____

Who completed this form? _____ Relationship to client: _____

Educational Background:

Individuals Living in the Home:

Presenting Problems and Reports of Consultation

Medical diagnosis of the voice problem (if known):

Current/past information on hearing (if known):

Presenting complaint:

Source: From Kenneth G. Shipley, *Systematic Assessment of Voice: Methods and Procedures for Evaluating Voice Disorders* (pp. 51-56). Copyright 1990 by and reprinted with permission of Academic Communication Associates, Oceanside, CA.

Description of the Voice Problem

Please check all that apply:

_____ too high in pitch   _____ strident voice
_____ too low in pitch   _____ harsh voice
_____ variable in pitch   _____ hoarse voice
_____ too loud   _____ quivering voice
_____ too soft or quiet   _____ tremor in the voice
_____ variable in loudness   _____ weak voice
_____ too nasal   _____ progressively weakening voice
_____ "stuffed up" quality (denasal)   _____ loss of voice
_____ breathy voice   _____ other (specify): _____
_____ shrill voice   _____

Voice History and Factors Associated with the Problem

When was the problem first noticed? By whom?

How does the voice differ from the voice of others who are the same age and gender?

How did the problem begin? (Suddenly? Over a period of time?)

Does the voice fluctuate or is it consistent?

What conditions or situations (specific environments, specific activities, time periods, etc.) seem to affect the voice?

Are there particular situations in which the voice seems to be the most troublesome? Least troublesome?

What limitations or problems have been experienced as a result of the voice problem?

How do other people react to the voice?

What do you feel may be causing or contributing to the voice problem?

In what ways do you feel the voice needs to be improved?

Is there any pain, irritation, or discomfort?

Has any previous therapy for the voice been provided? If so, what was done? Was it effective?

Description of the work environment (noisy machinery? dusty? smoky? etc.):

Description of the home environment (noisy? tense? competitive? smoky? etc.):

Medical History

Has a physician been seen because of the voice problem? What was found?

Recent medical treatments and hospitalizations:

Medications being taken currently:

Please check and describe all of the following that apply:

Comments:

____ accidents	_____
____ allergies	_____
____ asthma	_____
____ colds/bronchitis	_____
____ diabetes	_____
____ emotional difficulties	_____
____ headaches	_____
____ hearing difficulties	_____
____ laryngitis	_____
____ middle ear difficulties	_____
____ stress/tension	_____
____ surgical operations	_____
____ ulcers	_____
____ other: _____	_____

Lifestyle Factors

Please check any that apply, and describe any problems relevant to use of the voice:

Comments:

_____ arguing

_____ caffeine (sodas, coffee, etc.)

_____ crying

_____ inhalant usage

_____ laughing excessively

_____ public speaking

_____ screaming

_____ singing

_____ talking frequently

_____ talking at work

_____ talking over noise

_____ teaching

_____ throat clearing

_____ use of alcohol

_____ use of tobacco

_____ yelling

_____ other: _____

Climate and Environment-Related Considerations

Please check and describe any of the following that may apply. Weather, working, and home life situations should be considered.

Comments:

_____ cold

_____ dry

_____ heat

_____ pollen

_____ pollutants (e.g., smog)

_____ wind

_____ other: _____

Effects of Stress

Please describe any stressful situations that might affect the voice.

Situations at school or work:

Situations in the home or with the family:

Other conditions or activities:

APPENDIX C

BACKGROUND INFORMATION QUESTIONNAIRE
[FOR LINGUISTICALLY AND CULTURALLY DIVERSE CHILDREN]

This questionnaire can be used during a parent interview to collect information about the child's health, development, and educational background.

Instructions: We are going to ask you some questions about your child's medical history, educational background, and related areas. Please be as thorough as you can in your remarks. If I am not clear, please stop me and ask me to say it again. If you don't feel comfortable in answering the question, please let me know. All we want to do here is to obtain as much background information as possible, and, since you are the child's parent, we feel that you have much to contribute.

1. When was your child born? _____
2. Was this at a hospital? _____
3. How was the pregnancy? _____ How was your health during pregnancy? _____
4. How was the delivery? _____
5. Were any instruments used? _____
6. Were there any postnatal complications? _____
7. How was your child's physical development? _____

   Were there any handicapping conditions? _____ If yes, who made the diagnosis? _____ When? _____ How did you feel about it? _____

8. Was your child ever hospitalized? _____ If yes, where? _____ Who was the physician? _____
9. Were there problems in feeding? _____
10. Were there any prolonged illnesses? _____ High fever? _____ Accidents? _____
11. Has his/her hearing been checked? _____
12. Has his/her vision been checked? _____
13. Has he/she seen a dentist? _____ What is the condition of his/her teeth? _____

Source: From L. Lilly Cheng, *Assessing Asian Language Performance: Guidelines for Evaluating Limited-English Proficient Students* (2d ed.), pp. 165-167. Copyright 1991 by and reprinted with permission of Academic Communication Associates, Oceanside, CA.

14. What is his/her diet history? _____

_____

15. How is his/her diet now? _____

16. Does he/she have a pediatrician? _____ Who? _____
Has your child seen any other medical specialist? _____ If yes, who?
_____ When? _____ Where? _____
_____ Why? _____

17. When did you come to the United States? _____ Why did you come?

_____

For refugees: Was he/she ever in a refugee camp? _____ How long? _____
Tell us about it: _____

_____

18. Was he/she ever on a boat? _____ How long? _____ Tell us
about it: _____

_____

19. How many brothers and sisters does he/she have? _____ Are they all
here? _____

20. Are there any family members who had or have difficulty in speaking or hearing or
problems such as mental retardation, cerebral palsy, cleft palate, or stuttering? _____
If yes, please explain: _____

_____

21. Was your child ever in school? _____ Where? _____
How long? _____

22. How was his/her performance in school? _____
Grade? _____

23. Do you have a report from the school? _____ Any comments from the
teacher? _____

24. Was he/she involved in special programs? _____ How did he/she do?

_____

25. Was he/she in a day-care or child-care program? _____ If so, how did
he/she do? _____

26. Did he/she repeat a grade? _____ If yes, why? _____

_____

27. How was the program similar to his/her program now? _____
How was the program different from his/her program now? _____

_____

28. How many are living in your home? _____

29. Who takes care of your child after school? _____

30. Who makes the decisions at home? _____

31. Does your child have his/her own room? _____ If no, who does your child share the room with? _____ Where does he/she study? _____

32. Does your child mostly play inside the house? _____ Outside? _____
By himself/herself? _____ With a sibling? _____

33. Who does he/she play with? _____
Are they older or younger? _____
How does he/she play? _____

34. What does he/she like to play? _____
What toys do you have? _____
Does he/she read? _____ What books and magazines do you have? _____
_____

35. Do you work? _____ If yes, what do you do? _____
When are you home? _____

36. Does your spouse work? _____ If yes, what does he/she do?_____
When is he/she home? _____

37. What is your educational background? _____

38. What language(s) is used at home? _____

39. When did your child say his/her first word? _____
How do you feel about his/her speech now? _____

40. Do you feel that your child understands everything you say? _____
Explain: _____

41. Do you help your child with homework? _____

42. Does your child speak your native language with siblings? _____
Friends? _____

43. Do your children speak your native language or English among themselves? _____

44. Do you help your child with homework? _____

45. How do you feel about his/her maintenance of your native language? _____
_____

46. Do you send him/her to language school during the weekend? _____
What do you expect the school to do for your child? _____

47. Do you attend any social functions? _____ Where? _____
With whom? _____
What are your leisure activities? _____

48. Do you have difficulty disciplining your child? _____
His/her siblings? _____

49. What responsibilities are placed on your child? _____
_____

On his/her siblings? _____

50. Does he/she dress himself/herself? _____

51. Does he/she know your telephone number and address? _____

52. Do you read to him/her? _____   What are his/her favorite stories? _____

    _____

    Can he/she tell the story back to you? _____

53. Does he/she watch TV? _____   What is his/her favorite program? _____

    _____

54. Do you think your child is a hard worker? _____   If so, why? _____

    _____

    Do you think your child is lazy? _____   If so, why? _____

    _____

References

Abdrabbah, B. (1984). *Saudi Arabia: Forces of modernization.* Brattleboro, VT: Amana Books.

Allen, J., McNeill, E., & Schmidt, V. (1992). *Cultural awareness for children.* Menlo Park, CA: Addison-Wesley.

American Speech-Language-Hearing Association (1988, August). Inside the national office: Office of minority concerns. *Asha,* 30(8), 23-25.

American Speech-Language-Hearing Association (1990). Scope of practice, Speech-language pathology and audiology. *Asha,* 32 (Supplement 2), 1-2.

American Speech-Language-Hearing Association (1992, May). Our multicultural agenda: We're serious. *Asha,* 34, 38-39.

American Speech-Language-Hearing Association (1993, March). Preferred practice patterns for the professions of speech-language pathology and audiology. *Asha,* 35 (Supplement 11), 1-102.

American Speech-Language-Hearing Association (1994, March). Professional liability and risk management for the audiology and speech-language pathology professions. *Asha,* 36 (Supplement 12), 25-38.

American Speech-Language-Hearing Association (1995a, May). Special interest division—multiculturalism: Which language? *Asha,* 37, 26-27.

American Speech-Language-Hearing Association (1995b, March). Code of Ethics—1995. *Asha,* 37, 74-75.

Amidon, E. (1965). A technique for analyzing counselor–counselee interaction. In J. F. Adams (Ed.), *Counseling and guidance: A summary view* (pp. 50-56). New York: Macmillan.

Anderson, N. B. (1992). Understanding cultural diversity. *American Journal of Speech-Language Pathology,* 1(2), 11-12.

Anderson, P. P., & Fenichel, E. S. (1989). *Serving culturally diverse families of infants and toddlers with disabilities.* Washington, DC: National Center for Clinical Infant Programs.

Andrews, J. R., & Andrews, M. A. (1990). *Family based treatment in communicative disorders: A systemic approach.* Sandwich, IL: Janelle Publications.

Arambula, G. (1992). Acquired neurological disabilities in Hispanic adults. In H. Langdon (with L. L. Cheng) (Ed.), *Hispanic children and adults with communication disorders: Assessment and intervention* (pp. 373-407). Gaithersburg, MD: Aspen.

Atkins, D. V. (1994). Counseling children with hearing loss and their families. In J. G. Clark & F. N. Martin (Eds.), *Effective counseling in audiology: Perspectives and practice* (pp. 116-146). Englewood Cliffs, NJ: Prentice-Hall.

Barbara, D. A. (1958). *The art of listening.* Springfield, IL: Charles C Thomas.

Battle, D. (Ed.). (1993a). *Communication disorders in multicultural populations.* Stoneham, MA: Andover Medical Publishers.

Battle, D. (1993b). Introduction. In D. Battle (Ed.), *Communication disorders in multicultural populations* (pp. xv-xxiv). Stoneham, MA: Andover Medical Publishers.

Bebout, L., & Arthur, B. (1992). Cross-cultural attitudes about speech disorders. *Journal of Speech and Hearing Research, 35,* 45-52.

Benjamin, A. (1981). *The helping interview* (3d ed.). Boston: Houghton Mifflin.

Biggs, D., & Blocher, D. (1987). *Foundations of ethical counseling.* New York: Springer.

Bingham, W., Moore, D., & Gustad, J. (1959). *How to interview* (2d ed.). New York: Harper Brothers.

Bloom, C. M., & Cooperman, D. K. (1992). *The clinical interview: A guide for speech-language pathologists and audiologists* (2d ed.). Rockville, MD: National Student Speech-Language-Hearing Association.

Bondurant-Utz, J. A. (1994). Cultural diversity. In J. A. Bondurant-Utz & L. B. Luciano, *A practical guide to infant and preschool assessment in special education* (pp. 73-98). Boston: Allyn and Bacon.

Boone, D. R., & Prescott, T. (1972). Content and sequence analysis of speech and hearing therapy. *Asha, 14,* 58-62.

Bouty, A. (1992, Summer). Blackfeet to develop alphabet. *Newsletter of the National Association for Multicultural Education, 2*(1), 5.

Brammer, L. M. (1993). *The helping relationship: Processes and skills* (5th ed.). Boston: Allyn and Bacon.

Brammer, L. M., Abrego, P. J., & Shostrom, E. L. (1993). *Therapeutic counseling and psychotherapy* (6th ed.). Englewood Cliffs, NJ: Prentice-Hall.

Bramson, R. M. (1988). *Coping with difficult people.* New York: Dell.

Brigham Young University (1992). *Culturegrams.* Provo, UT: David M. Kennedy Center for International Studies.

Brown, D., & Brown, S. (1975). Procedures for behavioral consultation. *Elementary School Guidance and Counseling, 10,* 95-102.

Buell, L. H. (1985). *Understanding the immigrant Iraqi.* San Diego: Los Amigos Research Associates.

Burgoon, J. K. (1994). Nonverbal signals. In M. L. Knapp & G. R. Miller (Eds.), *Handbook of interpersonal communication* (2d ed.) (pp. 229-285). Thousand Oaks, CA: Sage Publications.

Campbell, I. C. (1989). *A history of the Pacific Islands.* Berkeley, CA: University of California Press.

Campbell, M. (1993, June-July). Teams and teamwork: Parental perspectives. *Asha, 35,* 32-33.

Casciani, J. M. (1978). Influence of models' race and sex on interviewees' self-disclosure. *Journal of Counseling Psychology, 215,* 435-440.

Chan, S. (1992a). Families with Filipino roots. In E. W. Lynch & M. J. Hanson (Eds.), *Developing cross-cultural competence: A guide to working with young children and their families* (pp. 259-300). Baltimore: Paul H. Brookes.

Chan, S. (1992b). Families with Asian roots. In E. W. Lynch & M. J. Hanson (Eds.),

Developing cross-cultural competence: A guide to working with young children and their families (pp. 181-257). Baltimore: Paul H. Brookes.

Cheng, L. L. (1987). Cross-cultural and linguistic considerations in working with Asian populations. *Asha*, 29(6), 33-37.

Cheng, L. L. (1989). Service delivery to Asian/Pacific LEP children: A cross-cultural framework. In K. G. Butler (Ed.), *Cross-cultural perspectives in language assessment and intervention* (pp. 181-194). Gaithersburg, MD: Aspen.

Cheng, L. L. (1991). *Assessing Asian language performance* (2d ed.). Oceanside, CA: Academic Communication Associates.

Cheng, L. L. (1993). Asian-American cultures. In D. Battle (Ed.), *Communication disorders in multicultural populations* (pp. 38-77). Stoneham, MA: Andover Medical Publishers.

Cheng, L. L., & Butler, K. (1993, March). Difficult discourse: Designing connection to deflect language impairment. Paper presented at the Annual Convention of the California Speech-Language-Hearing Association. Palm Springs, CA.

Cheng, L. L., & Damico, J. S. (1994, July). Strategies that work best. Paper presented at the Conference on Culturally Competent Assessment and Intervention with Hispanic and Asian/Pacific Islander Populations, Maui, HI.

Cheng, L. L., & Hammer, C. S. (1992). *Cultural perspectives of disabilities.* San Diego: Los Amigos Research Associates.

Cheng, L. L., & Ima, K. (1989). *Understanding the immigrant Pacific Islander.* San Diego: Los Amigos Research Associates.

Clark, J. G. (1994a). Audiologists' counseling purview. In J. C. Clark & F. N. Martin (Eds.), *Effective counseling in audiology: Perspectives and practice* (pp. 1-17). Englewood Cliffs, NJ: Prentice-Hall.

Clark, J. G. (1994b). Understanding, building, and maintaining relationships with patients. In J. C. Clark & F. N. Martin (Eds.), *Effective counseling in audiology: Perspectives and practice* (pp. 18-37). Englewood Cliffs, NJ: Prentice-Hall.

Clark, J. G., & Martin, F. N. (Eds.). (1994). *Effective counseling in audiology: Perspectives and practice.* Englewood Cliffs, NJ: Prentice-Hall.

Clarke, P. A. (1968). *Child-adolescent psychology.* Columbus, OH: Merrill.

Clemes, S., & D'Andrea, V. (1965). Patients' anxiety as a function of expectation and degree of initial interview ambiguity. *Journal of Consulting Psychology*, 29, 397-404.

Cohen, D., & Speken, R. H. (1985). Interviewing older adults. In A. Tolor (Ed.), *Effective interviewing* (pp. 118-135). Springfield, IL: Charles C Thomas.

Colton, R. H., & Casper, J. K. (1990). *Understanding voice problems: A physiological perspective for diagnosis and treatment.* Baltimore: Williams & Wilkins.

Cormier, L. S., & Hackney, H. (1987). *The professional counselor: A process guide to helping.* Englewood Cliffs, NJ: Prentice-Hall.

Cozad, R. L. (1974). *The speech clinician and the hearing impaired child.* Springfield, IL: Charles C Thomas.

Crais, E. R. (1991). Moving from "parent involvement" to family-centered services. *American Journal of Speech-Language Pathology*, 1(1), 5-8.

Culatta, R., & Goldberg, S. (1995). *Stuttering therapy: An integrated approach to theory and practice.* Boston: Allyn and Bacon.

Culpepper, B., Mendel, L. L., & McCarthy, P. A. (1994, June/July). Counseling experience and training offered by ESB-accredited programs. *Asha*, 36, 55-58.

Cunningham, C., & Davis, H. (1985). *Working with parents.* Philadelphia: Open University Press.

Dainow, S., & Bailey, C. (1988). *Developing skills with people: Training for person-to-person client contact.* New York: Wiley.

Dana, R. H. (1993). *Multicultural assessment perspectives for professional psychology.* Boston: Allyn and Bacon.

Darley, F. L. (1978). The case history. In F. L. Darley & D. C. Spriestersbach, *Diagnostic methods in speech pathology* (2d ed.) (pp. 37-96). New York: Harper & Row.

DeBlassie, R. R. (1976). *Counseling with Mexican American youth: Preconceptions and processes.* Austin, TX: Learning Concepts.

Dillard, J. M., & Reilly, R. R. (1988a). Introduction: A perspective on interviewing. In J. M. Dillard & R. R. Reilly (Eds.), *Systematic interviewing: Communication skills for professional effectiveness* (pp. 2-13). Columbus, OH: Merrill.

Dillard, J. M., & Reilly, R. R. (1988b). The professional: An introspection of self. In J. M. Dillard & R. R. Reilly (Eds.), *Systematic interviewing: Communication skills for professional effectiveness* (pp. 14-35). Columbus, OH: Merrill.

Dillard, J. M., & Reilly, R. R. (1988c). Communicative skills approach to interviewing. In J. M. Dillard & R. R. Reilly (Eds.), *Systematic interviewing: Communication skills for professional effectiveness* (pp. 36-65). Columbus, OH: Merrill.

Dillard, J. M., & Reilly, R. R. (Eds.). (1988d). *Systematic interviewing: Communication skills for professional effectiveness.* Columbus, OH: Merrill.

Dittman, A. T. (1987). The role of body movement in communication. In A. W. Siegman & S. Feldstein (Eds.), *Nonverbal behavior and communication* (2d. ed.) (pp. 37-64). Hillsdale, NJ: Lawrence Erlbaum Associates.

Donaghy, W. C. (1990). *The interview: Skills and applications.* Salem, WI: Sheffield.

Doster, J. (1972). Effects of instructions, modeling, and role rehearsal on interviewer behavior. *Journal of Consulting Psychology,* 39, 202-209.

Drapela, V. J. (1983). *The counselor as consultant and supervisor.* Springfield, IL: Charles C Thomas.

Edinburg, G. M., Zinberg, N. E., & Kelman, W. (1975). *Clinical interviewing and counseling: Principles and techniques.* New York: Appleton-Century-Crofts.

Edinger, J., & Patterson, M. (1983). Nonverbal involvement and social control. *Psychological Bulletin,* 93, 30-56.

Eisenberg, S., & Patterson, L. E. (1991). *Helping clients with special concerns.* Prospect Heights, IL: Waveland Press.

Emerick, L. (1969). *The parent interview.* Danville, IL: Interstate Publishers & Printers.

Emerick, L. L., & Hatten, J. T. (1979). *Diagnosis and evaluation in speech pathology* (2d ed.). Englewood Cliffs, NJ: Prentice-Hall.

Emerick, L. L., & Haynes, W. O. (1986). *Diagnosis and evaluation in speech pathology* (3d ed.). Englewood Cliffs, NJ: Prentice-Hall.

Enelow, A. J., & Swisher, S. N. (1986). *Interviewing and patient care* (3d ed.). New York: Oxford University Press.

Engelkes, J. R., & Vandergoot, D. (1982). *Introduction to counseling.* Boston: Houghton Mifflin.

Erickson, C. E. (1950). *The counseling interview.* New York: Prentice-Hall.

Ethridge, J. M. (1990). *China's unfinished revolution.* San Francisco: China Books & Periodicals.

Fenlason, A. F. (1962). *Essentials in interviewing.* New York: Harper & Row.

Fillmore, L. Wong (1993, February). Educating citizens for a multicultural society: The roles, responsibilities, and risks. Presentation at the National Association for Multicultural Education, Los Angeles.

Fitzgerald, L. (1995). English-as-a-second language learners' cognitive reading processes: A review of research in the United States. *Review of Educational Research,* 65(2), 145-190.

Fitzgerald, M. H., & Barker, J. C. (1993). Rehabilitation services for the Pacific. *The Western Journal of Medicine,* 59, 50-55.

Fretz, B. (1966). Postural movement in a counseling dyad. *Journal of Counseling Psychology,* 13, 335–343.

Freud, A. (1967). *The ego and the mechanisms of defense* (rev. ed.). New York: International Universities Press.

Gall, S. B., & Gall, T. L. (1993). *Statistical record of Asian Americans.* Detroit: Gale Research.

Garrett, A. (1982). *Interviewing: Its principles and methods* (3d ed.). New York: Family Service Association of America.

Gelso, C. J., & Karl, N. J. (1974). Perceptions of "counselors" and other help givers: What's in a label? *Journal of Counseling Psychology,* 21, 243–247.

Gerber, S. E. (1990). Prevention: *The etiology of communicative disorders in children.* Englewood Cliffs, NJ: Prentice-Hall.

Giles, H., & Street, R. L., Jr. (1994). Communicator characteristics and behavior. In M. L. Knapp & G. R. Miller (Eds.), *Handbook of interpersonal communication* (2d ed.) (pp. 103–161). Thousand Oaks, CA: Sage Publications.

Gilliland, H. (1992). *Teaching the Native American* (2d ed.). Dubuque: IA: Kendall/Hunt.

Goldberg, S. A. (1993). *Clinical intervention: A philosophy and methodology for clinical practice.* New York: Merrill.

Goldstein, A. P., & Higginbotham, H. N. (1991). Relationship-enhancement methods. In F. H. Kanfer & A. P. Goldstein (Eds.), *Helping people change: A textbook of methods* (4th ed.) (pp. 20–69). New York: Pergamon Press.

Green, S. W., & Perlman, S. M. (1995). Multicultural education and culture change: An anthropological perspective. *National Association of Multicultural Education,* 2(4), 4–6.

Gregory, H. H. (1995). Analysis and commentary. *Language, Speech, and Hearing Services in Schools,* 26(2), 196–200.

Hackney, H., & Cormier, L. S. (1979). *Counseling strategies and interventions* (2d ed.). Englewood Cliffs, NJ: Prentice-Hall.

Hackney, H., & Cormier, L. S. (1994). *Counseling strategies and interventions* (4th ed.). Boston: Allyn and Bacon.

Hall, E. (1964). Silent assumptions in social communication. *Disorders of Communication,* 42, 41–55.

Hamayan, E., & Damico, J. (1991). *Limiting bias in the assessment of bilingual students.* Austin, TX: Pro-Ed.

Hammer, C. S. (1994). Working with families of Chamorro and Carolinian cultures. *American Journal of Speech-Language Pathology,* 3(3), 5–12.

Hanline, M. F., & Daley, S. E. (1992). Family coping strategies and strengths in Hispanic, African-American, and Caucasian families of young children. *Topics in Early Childhood Special Education,* 12(3), 351–366.

Hanson, M. J. (1992). Ethnic, cultural, and language diversity in intervention settings. In E. W. Lynch & M. J. Hanson (Eds.), *Developing cross-cultural competence: A guide for working with young children and their families* (pp. 3–18). Baltimore: Paul H. Brookes.

Harris, G. (1993). American Indian cultures: A lesson in diversity. In D. Battle (Ed.), *Communication disorders in multicultural populations* (pp. 78–113). Stoneham, MA: Andover Medical Publishers.

Hartbauer, R. E. (1978). Counseling the uninformed and misinformed. In R. E. Hartbauer (Ed.), *Counseling in communicative disorders* (pp. 107–122). Springfield, IL: Charles C Thomas.

Hayes-Bautista, D. E., Hurtado, A., Valdez, R. B., & Hernandez, A. C. R. (1992). *No longer a minority: Latinos and social policy in California.* Los Angeles: Chicano Studies Research Center, University of California.

Haynes, W. O., Pindzola, R. H., & Emerick, L. L. (1992). *Diagnosis and evaluation in speech pathology* (4th ed.). Englewood Cliffs, NJ: Prentice-Hall.

Hegde, M. N. (1993). *Treatment procedures in communicative disorders* (2d ed.). Austin, TX: Pro-Ed.

Hegde, M. N. (1994). *Clinical research in communicative disorders: Principles and strategies* (2d ed.). Austin, TX: Pro-Ed.

Hegde, M. N. (1995). *Introduction to communicative disorders* (2d ed.). Austin, TX: Pro-Ed.

Hegde, M. N., & Davis, D. (1995). *Clinical methods and practicum in speech-language pathology* (2d ed.). San Diego: Singular Publishing Group.

Henry, W. A. (1990, April). Beyond the melting pot. *Time Magazine,* 135(15), 28–31.

Horton, C. P., & Smith, J. C. (Eds.). (1993). *Statistical record of Black America* (2d ed.). Detroit: Gale Research.

Hutchinson, B. B. (1979). Dialogues: Client-centered communication. In B. B. Hutchinson, M. L. Hanson, & M. J. Mecham (Eds.), *Diagnostic handbook of speech pathology* (pp. 1–29). Baltimore: Williams & Wilkins.

Hutchinson, B. B., Hanson, M. L., & Mecham, M. J. (Eds.). (1979). *Diagnostic handbook of speech pathology.* Baltimore: Williams & Wilkins.

Ima K., & Cheng, L. L. (1989). *Understanding the refugee Hmong.* San Diego: Los Amigos Research Associates.

Irujo, S. (1988). An introduction of intercultural differences and similarities in nonverbal communication. In J. S. Wurzel (Ed.), *Toward multiculturalism* (pp. 142–150). Yarmouth, ME: Intercultural Press.

Irwin, R. B. (1969). *Speech and hearing therapy: Clinical and educational principles and practices.* Pittsburgh: Stanwix House.

Ivey, A. E. (1983). *Intentional interviewing and counseling: Facilitating client development.* Monterey, CA: Brooks/Cole.

Ivey, A. E. (1994). *Intentional interviewing and counseling: Facilitating client development in a multicultural society* (3d ed.). Pacific Grove, CA: Brooks/Cole.

Joe, J. R., & Malach, R. S. (1992). Families with Native American roots. In E. W. Lynch & M. J. Hanson (Eds.), *Developing cross-cultural competence: A guide to working with young children and their families* (pp. 89–119). Baltimore: Paul H. Brookes.

John-Roger, & McWilliams, P. (1992). *The portable Life 101.* Los Angeles: Prelude Press.

Johns, G. (1975). Effects of informational order and frequency of applicant evaluation upon linear information processing competence of interviewers. *Journal of Applied Psychology,* 60, 427–433.

Johnson, C. D. (1994). Educational consultation: Talking with parents and school personnel. In J. G. Clark & F. N. Martin (Eds.), *Effective counseling in audiology: Perspectives and practice* (pp. 184–209). Englewood Cliffs, NJ: Prentice-Hall.

Johnson, R. (1988). Interviewing adults. In J. M. Dillard & R. R. Reilly (Eds.), *Systematic interviewing: Communication skills for professional effectiveness* (pp. 140–159). Columbus, OH: Merrill.

Jones, S. D. (1993). Communicating with parents and teachers. In R. L. Lowe (Ed.), *Speech-language pathology and related professions in the schools* (pp. 241–260). Boston: Allyn and Bacon.

Jung, J. H. (1989). *Genetic syndromes in communication disorders.* Boston: College-Hill Press.

Kanfer, F., Phillips, J., Matarazzo, J., & Saslow, G. (1960). Experimental modification of interviewer content in standardized interviews. *Journal of Consulting Psychology,* 24, 528–536.

Kayser, H. (1993). Hispanic cultures. In D. Battle (Ed.), *Communication disorders in multicultural populations* (pp. 114–157). Stoneham, MA: Andover Medical Publishers.

Keane, T. M., & Verman, S. H. (1985). The behavioral interview: Searching for clues to effective behavioral change. In A. Tolor (Ed.), *Effective interviewing* (pp. 21–49). Springfield, IL: Charles C Thomas.

Keefe, S. E. (1988). *Appalachian mental health.* Lexington: University Press of Kentucky.

Kennedy, E. (1977). *On becoming a counselor: A basic guide for non-professional counselors.* New York: Seabury Press.

Kennedy, E., & Charles, S. C. (1990). *On becoming a counselor: A basic guide for nonprofessional counselors* (rev. ed.). New York: Continuum Press.

Kinney, J., & Leaton, G. (1991). *Loosening the grip: A handbook of alcohol information* (4th ed.). St. Louis: Mosby-Year Book.

Kinzie, J. D., Sack, W., Angell, R., Clarke, G., & Ben, R. (1989). A three-year follow-up study of Cambodian young people traumatized as children. *Journal of American Academy of Child Psychiatry, 28*(4), 501–504.

Kleinke, C. L. (1986). *Meeting and understanding people.* New York: W. H. Freeman.

Kleinke, C., Staneski, R., & Berger, D. (1975). Evaluation of an interviewer as a function of interviewer gaze, reinforcement of subject gaze, and interviewer attractiveness. *Journal of Personality and Social Psychology, 31,* 115–122.

Knapp, M. L. (1972). *Nonverbal communication in human interaction.* New York: Holt, Rinehart & Winston.

Knapp, M. L., & Hall, J. A. (1992). *Nonverbal communication in human interaction* (3d. ed.). New York: Holt, Rinehart, & Winston.

Kottler, J. A. & Blau, D. S. (1989). *The imperfect therapist: Learning from failure in therapeutic practice.* San Francisco: Jossey-Bass.

Kozloff, M. A. (1994). *Improving educational outcomes for children with disabilities.* Baltimore: Paul H. Brookes.

Kroth, R. L. (1985). *Communicating with parents of exceptional children* (2d ed.). Denver: Love Publishing. (Excerpts in chapters used with permission.)

Krumboltz, J. D., & Thoresen, C. E. (1969). The effect of behavioral counseling in group and individual settings on information-seeking behavior. *Journal of Counseling Psychology, 11,* 324–333.

Kübler-Ross, E. (1969). *On death and dying.* Englewood Cliffs, NJ: Prentice-Hall.

Kübler-Ross, E. (1986). *Death, the final stage of growth.* New York: Touchstone.

Lane, V. W., & Molyneaux, D. (1992). *The dynamics of communicative development.* Englewood Cliffs, NJ: Prentice-Hall.

Lang, G., van der Molen, H., Trower, P., & Look, R. (1990). *Personal conversations: Roles and skills for counsellors.* London: Routledge.

Langdon, H. W. (with Cheng, L. L.) (1992). *Hispanic children and adults with communication disorders: Assessment and intervention.* Gaithersburg, MD: Aspen.

Larson, V. Lord, & McKinley, N. (1995). *Language disorders in older students.* Eau Claire, WI: Thinking Publications.

Lavorato, A. S., & McFarlane, S. C. (1988). Counseling clients with voice disorders. *Seminars in Speech and Language, 9,* 237–255. (Excerpts in Chapters 9 and 10 used with permission of the authors.)

Lee, C. C., & Richardson, B. L. (Eds.). (1991). *Multicultural issues in counseling: New approaches to diversity.* Alexandria, VA: American Association for Counseling and Development.

Leigh, J. E., & Marshall, S. (1983). Counseling the disabled and their parents: A review of the literature. In L. Buscaglia (Ed.), *The disabled and their parents: A counseling challenge* (rev. ed.) (pp. 35–60). Thorofare, NJ: Slack, Inc.

Leith, W. R. (1993). *Clinical methods in communication disorders* (2d ed.). Austin: TX: Pro-Ed.

Leslie, L. A. (1992). The role of informal support networks in the adjustment of Central American immigrant families. *Journal of Community Psychology, 20*(3), 243–256.

Lewis, J., & Vang, L. (1987). *The Hmong language: Sounds and alphabets—Indochinese Refugee Education Guide.* Arlington, VA: Center for Applied Linguistics.

Libby, W., & Yaklevich, D (1973). Personality determinants of eye contact and direction of gaze aversion. *Journal of Personal and Social Psychology, 27,* 197–206.

Long, S. O. (1992). *Japan: A country study.* Washington, DC: Department of the Army.

Lund, N. J., & Duchan, J. F. (1993). *Assessing children's language in naturalistic contexts* (3d ed.). Englewood Cliffs, NJ: Prentice-Hall.

Luterman, D. M. (1991). *Counseling the communicatively disordered and their families* (2d ed.). Austin, TX: Pro-Ed.

Lynch, E. W., & Hanson, M. J. (Eds.). (1992a). *Developing cross-cultural competence: A guide for working with young children and their families.* Baltimore: Paul H. Brookes.

Lynch, E. W., & Hanson, M. J. (1992b). Steps in the right direction: Implications for interventionists. In E. W. Lynch & M. J. Hanson (Eds.), *Developing cross-cultural competence: A guide for working with young children and their families* (pp. 355–369). Baltimore: Paul H. Brookes.

MacLean, D., & Gould, S. (1988). *The helping process: An introduction.* New York: Croom Helm.

Maestas, A. G., & Erickson, J. G. (1992). Mexican immigrant mothers' beliefs about disabilities. *American Journal of Speech-Language Pathology, 1,* 5–10.

Martin, F. N. (1994). Conveying diagnostic information. In J. G. Clark & F. N. Martin (Eds.), *Effective counseling in audiology: Perspectives and practice* (pp. 38–69). Englewood Cliffs, NJ: Prentice-Hall.

Martin, J., & Hiebert, B. A. (1985). *Instructional counseling: A method for counselors.* Pittsburgh: University of Pittsburgh Press.

Matsuda, M. (1989). Working with Asian parents: Some communication strategies. *Topics in Language Disorders, 9,* 45–53.

Matsuda, M., & O'Connor, L. (1993, March). Creating an effective partnership: Training bilingual communication aides. Paper presented at the Annual Convention of the California Speech-Language-Hearing Association, Palm Springs, CA.

Mattes, L., & Omark, D. (1991). *Speech and language assessment for the bilingual handicapped* (2d ed.). Oceanside, CA: Academic Communication Associates.

Matz, M. (1991). Helping families cope with grief. In S. Eisenberg & L. E. Patterson (Eds.), *Helping clients with special concerns* (pp. 213–238). Prospect Heights, IL: Waveland Press.

McCroskey, J. C., Richmond, V. P., & Stewart, R. A. (1986). *One on one: The foundations of interpersonal communication.* Englewood Cliffs, NJ: Prentice-Hall.

McDonald, E. T. (1962). *Understand those feelings.* Pittsburgh: Stanwix House.

McDonald, P. A., & Haney, M. (1988). *Counseling the older adult: A training manual in clinical gerontology* (2d ed.). Lexington, MA: Lexington Books.

McFarlane, S. C., Fujiki, M., & Brinton, B. (1984). *Coping with communicative handicaps: Resources for the practicing clinician.* San Diego, CA: College-Hill Press.

Mehrabian, A. (1968). Inference of attitudes from posture, orientation, and distance of a communicator. *Journal of Consulting and Clinical Psychology, 32,* 296–308.

Mehrabian, A. (1972). *Nonverbal communication.* Chicago: Aldine Atherton.

Meier, S. T. (1989). *The elements of counseling.* Pacific Grove, CA: Brooks/Cole.

Meier, S. T., & Davis, S. R. (1993). *The elements of counseling* (2d ed.). Pacific Grove, CA: Brooks/Cole.

Meitus, I. J., & Weinberg, B. (Eds.). (1983). *Diagnosis in speech-language pathology.* Baltimore: University Park Press.

Merriam-Webster Collegiate Dictionary (10th ed.) (1993). Springfield, MA: Merriam-Webster, Inc.

Mitchell, C. J. (1988). Counseling for the parent. In R. J. Roeser & M. P. Downs (Eds.), *Auditory disorders in school children* (2d ed.) (pp. 350-364). New York: Theime Medical Publishers.

Mokuau, N., & Tauili'ili, P. (1992). Families with Native Hawaiian and Pacific Island roots. In E. W. Lynch & M. J. Hanson (Eds.), *Developing cross-cultural competence: A guide for working with young children and their families* (pp. 301-318). Baltimore: Paul H. Brookes.

Molyneaux, D., & Lane, V. W. (1982). *Effective interviewing: Techniques and analysis.* Boston: Allyn and Bacon.

Montgomery, J. K., & Herer, G. (1994). Future watch: Our schools in the 21st century. *Language, Speech, and Hearing Services in Schools,* 25(3), 130-135.

Moses, K. L. (1985). Dynamic intervention with families. In E. Cherow (Ed.), *Hearing-impaired children and youth with developmental disabilities* (pp. 82-98), Washington, DC: Gallaudet College Press.

Moursund, J. (1985). *The process of counseling and therapy.* Englewood Cliffs, NJ: Prentice-Hall.

Moursund, J. (1993). *The process of counseling and therapy* (3d ed.). Englewood Cliffs, NJ: Prentice-Hall.

Mowrer, D. (1977). *Methods of modifying speech behaviors: Learning theory in speech pathology.* Columbus, OH: Merrill.

Mowrer, D. E. (1988). *Methods of modifying speech behaviors: Learning theory in speech pathology* (2d ed.). Prospect Heights, IL: Waveland Press.

Nation, J. E., & Aram, D. M. (1991). *Diagnosis of speech and language disorders* (2d ed.). San Diego: Singular Publishing Group.

National Coalition of Hispanic Health and Human Service Organizations (1988). *Delivering preventive health care to Hispanics: A manual for providers.* Washington, DC: Author.

Neidecker, E. A., & Blosser, J. L. (1993). *School programs in speech-language: Organization and management* (3d ed.). Englewood Cliffs, NJ: Prentice-Hall.

Nellum-Davis, P. (1993). Clinical practice issues. In D. Battle (Ed.), *Communication disorders in multicultural populations.* Stoneham, MA: Andover Medical Publishers.

Nicolosi, L., Harryman, E., & Kresheck, J. (1989). *Terminology of communicative disorders* (3d ed.). Baltimore: Williams & Wilkins.

Nirenberg, J. S. (1968). *Getting through to people.* Englewood Cliffs, NJ: Prentice-Hall.

Okun, B. F. (1992). *Effective helping: Interviewing and counseling techniques* (4th ed.). Pacific Grove, CA: Brooks/Cole.

Orr, D. W., & Adams, N. O. (1987). *Life cycle counseling: Guidelines for helping people.* Springfield, IL: Charles C Thomas.

Paniagua, F. A. (1994). *Assessing and treating culturally diverse clients.* Thousand Oaks: CA: Sage Publications.

Pannbacker, M., Middleton, G. F., & Vekovius, G. T. (1996). *Ethical practices in speech-language pathology and audiology: Case studies.* San Diego: Singular Publishing Group.

Paul-Brown, D. (1994, May). Clinical record keeping in audiology and speech-language pathology. *Asha*, 36, 40–42; 39.

Pederson, P. B. (Ed.). (1985). *Handbook of cross-cultural counseling and therapy.* Westport, CT: Greenwood Press.

Pederson, P. B., Draguns, J. G., Lonner, W. J., & Trimble, J. E. (Eds.). (1989). *Counseling across cultures* (3d ed.). Honolulu: University of Hawaii Press.

Pederson, P. B., & Ivey, A. (1993). *Culture-centered counseling and interviewing skills: A practical guide.* Westport, CT: Praeger.

Peterson, H. A., & Marquardt, T. P. (1990). *Appraisal and diagnosis of speech and language disorders* (2d ed.). Englewood Cliffs, NJ: Prentice-Hall.

Peterson, H. A., & Marquardt, T. P. (1994). *Appraisal and diagnosis of speech and language disorders* (3d ed.). Englewood Cliffs, NJ: Prentice-Hall.

Phillips, J., Matarazzo, R., Matarazzo, J., Saslow, G., & Kanfer, F. (1961). Relationships between descriptive content and interaction behavior in interviews. *Journal of Consulting Psychology*, 25, 260–266.

Powell, W., Jr. (1968). Differential effectiveness of interviewer interventions in an experimental interview. *Journal of Consulting and Clinical Psychology*, 32, 210–215.

Prescott, T., & Tesauro, P. (1974). A method for quantification and description of clinical interactions with aurally handicapped children. *Journal of Speech and Hearing Disorders*, 39, 234–243.

Purkey, W. W., & Schmidt, J. J. (1987). *The inviting relationship: An expanded perspective for professional counseling.* Englewood Cliffs, NJ: Prentice-Hall.

Rache, L., Bernstein, L., & Veenhuis, R. (1974). Evaluation of a systematic approach to teaching interviewing. *Journal of Medical Education*, 49, 589–595.

Rae, L. (1988). *The skills of interviewing: A guide for managers and trainers.* New York: Nichols.

Randall-David, E. (1989). *Strategies for working with culturally diverse communities and clients.* Washington, DC: Association for the Care of Children's Health.

Reilly, R. R. (1988). Stages of the interview process. In J. M. Dillard & R. R. Dillard (Eds.), *Systematic interviewing: Communication skills for professional effectiveness* (pp. 66–89). Columbus, OH: Merrill.

Resnick, D. M. (1993). *Professional ethics for audiologists and speech-language pathologists.* San Diego: Singular Publishing Group.

Reyes, B. (1994). Management of adult neurogenic patients: A multicultural perspective. In H. Kayser (Ed.), *Seminars in speech and language: Communicative impairments and bilingualism* (pp. 165–173). New York: Thieme Medical Publishers.

Rich, J. (1968). *Interviewing children and adolescents.* New York: Macmillan.

Richardson, S., Dohrenwend, B., & Klein, D. (1965). *Interviewing: Its form and function.* New York: Basic Books.

Rick, K., & Forward, J. (1992). Acculturation and perceived intergenerational differences among Hmong youth. *Journal of Cross-Cultural Psychology*, 23(1), 85–94.

Riley, F. T. (1972). The effects of seating arrangement in the dyadic interaction interview upon the perceptual evaluation of the counseling relationship among secondary students. *Dissertation Abstract International*, 33(4-A), 1447–1448.

Roberts, S. D., & Bouchard, K. R. (1989). Establishing rapport in rehabilitative audiology. *Journal of Aural Rehabilitative Audiology*, 22, 67–73.

Rogers, C. (1951). *Client-centered therapy.* Boston: Houghton Mifflin.

Rogers, C. (1986). In I. Kutash & A. Wold (Eds.), *Psychotherapist's casebook: Theory and technique in practice* (pp. 197–208). San Francisco: Jossey-Bass.

Rollin, W. J. (1987). *The psychology of communication disorders in individuals and their families.* Englewood Cliffs, NJ: Prentice-Hall.

Roseberry-McKibbin, C. A. (1994, August 8). Understanding the impact of immigrant/refugee status on clients. *Advance for Speech-Language Pathologists & Audiologists,* 4(16), 8–9.

Roseberry-McKibbin, C. (1995). *Multicultural students with special language needs: Practical strategies for assessment and intervention.* Oceanside, CA: Academic Communication Associates.

Rosenfeld, H. (1967). Nonverbal reciprocation of approval: An experimental analysis. *Journal of Experimental and Social Psychology,* 3, 102–111.

Rosenfeld, L. B., & Civikly, J. M. (1976). *With words unspoken: The nonverbal experience.* New York: Holt, Rinehart & Winston.

Ruiz, N. T. (1991). Effective instruction for language minority children with mild disabilities. *ERIC Digest,* EDO-ED-91-4, 11–12.

Samovor, L. A., & Hellweg, S. A. (1982). *Interviewing: A communicative approach.* Dubuque, IA: Gorsuch Scarisbrick.

Scheflen, A. (1964). The significance of posture in communication systems. *Psychiatry,* 27, 316–331.

Scheuerle, J. (1992). *Counseling in speech-language pathology and audiology.* New York: Merrill.

Schum, R. L. (1986). *Counseling in speech and hearing practice.* Rockville, MD: National Student Speech-Language-Hearing Association.

Schuyler, V., & Rushmer, N. (1987). *Parent-infant habilitation: A comprehensive approach to working with hearing-impaired infants and toddlers and their families.* Portland, OR: IHR [Infant Hearing Resource] Publications.

Sharifzadeh, V. S. (1992). Families with Middle Eastern roots. In E. W. Lynch & M. J. Hanson (Eds.), *Developing cross-cultural competence: A guide for working with young children and their families* (pp. 319–351). Baltimore: Paul H. Brookes.

Shertzer, B. & Stone, S. C. (1980). *Fundamentals of counseling* (3d ed.). Boston: Houghton Mifflin.

Shipley, K. G. (1990). *Systematic assessment of voice: Methods and procedures for evaluating voice disorders.* Oceanside, CA: Academic Communication Associates.

Shipley, K. G. (1992). *Interviewing and counseling in communicative disorders: Principles and procedures.* New York: Merrill.

Shipley, K. G., & McAfee, J. G. (1992). *Assessment in speech-language pathology: A resource manual.* San Diego: Singular Publishing Group.

Shipley, K. G., & Wood, J. M. (1996). *The elements of interviewing.* San Diego: Singular Publishing Group.

Siegman, A. W., & Feldstein, S. (Eds.). (1987). *Nonverbal behavior and communication* (2d ed.). Hillsdale, NJ: Lawrence Erlbaum Associates.

Silverman, F. H. (1993). *Research design and evaluation in speech-language pathology* (3d ed.). Englewood Cliffs, NJ: Prentice-Hall.

Smith, A. (1973). *Transracial communication.* Englewood Cliffs, NJ: Prentice-Hall.

Sobol, T. (1990). Understanding diversity. *Educational Leadership,* 48(3), 27–30.

Stemple, J. C. (1993). *Voice therapy: Clinical studies.* St. Louis: Mosby-Year Book.

Stewart, C. J. (1972). *Types and uses of questions in interviews: On speech communication.* New York: Holt, Rinehart & Winston.

Stewart, C. J., & Cash, W. B. (1978). *Interviewing: Principles and practices* (2d ed.). Dubuque, IA: William C. Brown.

Stewart, C. J., & Cash, W. B. (1994). *Interviewing: Principles and practices* (7th ed.). Dubuque, IA: William C. Brown.

Stone, J. R., & Olswang, L. B. (1989, June–July). The hidden challenge in counseling. *Asha,* 31, 27–31.

Sue, D. W. (1988). *Counseling the culturally different: Theory and practice* (2d ed.). New York: Wiley.

Sweeney, T. J. (1971). *Rural poor students and guidance.* Boston: Houghton Mifflin.

Tannen, D. (1994). *Talking from 9 to 5.* New York: William R. Morrow.

Tanner, D. C. (1980). Loss and grief: Implications for the speech-language pathologist. *Asha,* 22, 916–928.

Taylor, J. S. (1992). *Speech-language pathology services in the schools.* Boston: Allyn and Bacon.

Taylor, O. L., & Clarke, M. G. (1994). Culture and communication disorders: A theoretical framework. In H. Kayser (Ed.), *Seminars in speech and language: Communicative impairments and bilingualism* (pp. 103–114). New York: Thieme Medical Publishers.

Terrell, S. L., & Terrell, F. (1993). African-American cultures. In D. Battle (Ed.), *Communication disorders in multicultural populations* (pp. 3–37). Stoneham, MA: Andover Medical Publishers.

Thompson, J. (1973). *Beyond words.* New York: Citation Press.

Thornton, C. (1994, April 4). Empowering families of children with disabilities. *Advance for Speech-Language Pathologists & Audiologists,* 4(7), 8–9.

Tidwell, B. J., Kuumba, M. B., Jones, D. J., & Watson, B. C, (1993). Fast facts: African Americans in the 1990s. In B. Tidwell (Ed.), *The state of Black America, 1993* (pp. 243–265). New York: National Urban League.

Tiegerman-Farber, E. (1995). *Language and communication intervention in preschool children.* Boston: Allyn and Bacon.

Tomblin, J. B. (1994). Perspective on diagnosis. In J. B. Tomblin, H. L. Morris, & D. C. Spriestersbach (Eds.), *Diagnosis in speech-language pathology* (pp. 1–28). San Diego: Singular Publishing Group.

Tomblin, J. B., Morris, H. L., & Spriestersbach, D. C. (Eds.) (1994). *Diagnosis in speech-language pathology.* San Diego: Singular Publishing Group.

Trace, R. (1993, December 6). Support groups play vital role for patients and families. *Advance for Speech-Language Pathologists & Audiologists,* 2(25), 6–7.

Trace, R. (1995, July 10). Treating the patient with a substance abuse problem. *Advance for Speech-Language Pathologists & Audiologists,* 5(27), 9.

U.S. Bureau of the Census (1992). *Statistical Abstract of the United States, 1992* (112th ed.). Washington, DC: U.S. Government Printing Office.

Van Riper, C. (1966). Success and failure in speech therapy. *Journal of Speech and Hearing Disorders,* 31, 276–279.

Van Riper, C. (1979). *A career in speech pathology.* Englewood Cliffs, NJ: Prentice-Hall. (Excerpts in chapters used with permission.)

Wallace, G. L. (1993). Adult neurogenic disorders. In D. Battle (Ed.), *Communication disorders in multicultural populations* (pp. 239–255). Stoneham, MA: Andover Medical Publishers.

Wallace, G. L. (1994, July). Asian/Pacific Islander cultures. Paper presentation at the Conference on Culturally Competent Assessment and Intervention with Hispanic and Asian/Pacific Islander Populations, Maui, HI.

Walton, P. (1995). Whose "culture" are we talking about anyway? *National Association for Multicultural Education,* 2(4), 1.

Webster, E. (1966). Parent counseling by speech pathologists and audiologists. *Journal of Speech and Hearing Disorders,* 31, 331–340.

Webster, E. (1968). Procedures for group parent counseling in speech pathology and audiology. *Journal of Speech and Hearing Disorders,* 33, 127–131.

Webster, E. J., & Ward, L. M. (1993). *Working with parents of young children with disabilities.* San Diego: Singular Publishing Group.

Westby, C. E. (1990). Ethnographic interviewing: Asking the right questions to the right people in the right ways. *Journal of Childhood Communication Disorders,* 13, 101-111.

Westby, C. E., & Rouse, G. R. (1985). Culture in education and the instruction of language-learning disabled students. *Topics in Language Disorders,* 5(4), 15-28.

Willis, W. (1992). Families with African American roots. In E. W. Lynch & M. J. Hanson (Eds.), *Developing cross-cultural competence: A guide for working with young children and their families* (pp. 121-150). Baltimore: Paul H. Brookes.

Woody, R. H., Hansen, J. C., & Rossberg, R. H. (1989). *Counseling strategies and services.* Pacific Grove, CA: Brooks/Cole.

Woolf, G. (1971). Information specificity: A correlate of verbal output in the diagnostic interview. *Journal of Speech and Hearing Disorders,* 36, 518-526.

Zebrowski, P. M., & Schum, R. L. (1993). Counseling parents of children who stutter. *American Journal of Speech-Language Pathology,* 2(2), 65-73.

Zuniga, M. E. (1992). Families with Latino roots. In E. W. Lynch & M. J. Hanson (Eds.), *Developing cross-cultural competence: A guide to working with young children and their families* (pp. 151-179). Baltimore: Paul H. Brookes.

Index

Page numbers for names in reference section appear in italics.